7429

*Psychology and
mental health
nursing*

Psychology Applied to Nursing series

Titles in the series

Psychology and Mental Health Nursing   *Derek Milne*
Psychology of Nursing Care   *Neil Niven and Jill Robinson*
Psychology and Nursing Children   *Jo Douglas*

Psychology and mental health nursing

Derek Milne

Regional Tutor in Clinical Psychology,
Northumberland District Psychology Service and
the University of Newcastle upon Tyne

Series Editor: Professor Dave Müller
Consultant: Erica Joslyn

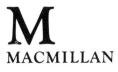

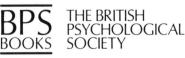

First published 1993 by
BPS Books (The British Psychological Society),
St. Andrews House, 48 Princess Road East, Leicester LE1 7DR
in association with
THE MACMILLAN PRESS LTD
Houndmills, Basingstoke, Hampshire RG21 2XS
and London
Companies and representatives
throughout the world

ISBN 0–333–58954–8
ISBN 0–333–57768–X

A catalogue record for this book is available
from the British Library

Typeset by Cambrian Typesetters, Frimley, Surrey
Printed in Hong Kong

In memory and recognition of my twin Dennis Milne,
who loved to communicate his
enthusiasm about his own subject

Contents

List of exercises

Series Editor's Foreword

This book series is designed for the nursing profession and those responsible for teaching nurses on both pre- and post-registration programmes of study. The linking of the nursing curriculum with higher education and the implementation of Project 2000 has led to a radical revision of nurse education. Many nurses on pre-registration courses will be studying at degree level and will be gaining an academic qualification as well as entry to the nursing Register. These forward looking and exciting changes have led to the need to develop new reading material for nurses to progress both academically and professionally.

This is equally true for those nurses post-registration who are committed to enhancing their qualifications base. The expansion in higher education has led to a wide range of part-time degree courses for nurses as well as the linking of post-registration courses such as health visiting and district nursing with higher level academic qualifications. The introduction by the English National Board for Nursing, Midwifery and Health Visiting of the Higher Award for experienced professionals is an important step to facilitate continuing professional development for the nursing profession. This, in turn, has led to the need to bring together nursing and those disciplines akin to professional practice.

It has long been recognized that the study of psychology in applied contexts is of major importance both in learning to become a nurse and in moving towards becoming a reflective practitioner. Psychology as the scientific study of human behaviour provides a methodology through which individuals can evaluate the effectiveness of the provision of care within hospitals and the community. Psychology and nursing are both characterized by adopting a scientific and hence an empirical approach to the collection of information and using it to make informed decisions. The importance of research within the fields of psychology and nursing has led to psychologists and nurses working together both in terms of curriculum design and in carrying out research to help provide high standards of patient care.

All the books in the series are characterized by the emphasis placed on the critical examination of research evidence. Each volume aims to review current practice from a psychological perspective in the light of current research being undertaken by nurses as well as other professionals. The authors, in bringing together this information, all seek to offer recommendations to inform nursing practice not in a prescriptive way but in a way in which nurses themselves can evaluate their practice. All the texts are ideal for students studying psychology and nursing for the first time and are written at the appropriate level for inclusion on reading lists for students studying at diploma and degree level. At the same time, the applied research nature of the texts makes them invaluable as a source to support nurses gaining further qualifications as part of their professional development.

The texts are contemporary, derived from a strong research base and written by authors with considerable experience of teaching nurses and working with them professionally. I hope that you enjoy this volume in the series and are attracted to the related texts which, taken together, provide nurses with a resource base from which to study psychology as applied to nursing.

Professor Dave Müller
Suffolk College, Ipswich   *24 September 1992*

Foreword

The publication of this book is timely in more ways than one. Mental health nursing has rarely been absent from one 'crossroads' or another over the past twenty years, and at present it stands at a very significant crossroads indeed. The level of critical analysis of mental health nursing, in various settings, with a wide range of people-with-problems-of-living, has never been greater. The range of theoretical explanations of mental health nursing has expanded exponentially, year by year. One model of caring competes with another, each vying for our attention like all *enfants terribles*. The establishment of Project 2000 branch programmes adds to this expansion, generating new educational and practice agendas. And yet, despite the research explosion and our promiscuous model-making, we appear no more certain of who we are and what, exactly, we are doing here. Our knowledge *about* mental health nursing is greater than ever; yet our understanding of what it *is*, seems no clearer.

The search for identity, long a feature of mental health nursing *angst*, is the crossroads to which we return with a saddening regularity, like travellers wearily tramping in circles. What does Derek Milne's text offer tomorrow's students, those charged with their preparation, or any other seekers after truth? This book should not be viewed as manna from heaven, or a transcription from the Oracle. Clearly this was not the author's intention. It does, however, offer much food for thought. The reader will be sustained by considerable exploration and clarification, some direction and numerous challenges; all presented sensitively and wisely. As a whole, the book is a timely reminder that caring and helping are not professional issues to be defined out of the person-in-care's hearing. Dr Milne reminds us that helping and caring are tied up, inextricably, with the *person* in care. He explores, with a fastidious curiosity, different views, and theoretical representations of the world of the 'patient': from the 'self' to the environment, taking account of relationships, values and customs along the way. It may be too soon to expect definitive answers about the nature of mental health nursing. This book does, however, offer a valuable vantage point from which we might gain a psychological perspective on the 'nurse–patient' relationship. I should add that it is an elevated view: one that raises the consciousness.

I believe that psychology is undoubtedly one of the 'pillars of wisdom' upon which effective mental health nursing might be built. This was not always the case. My own introduction to the subject was prefaced by the ignorant, though not uncommon, declaration that 'psychology is everything you ever knew, in language you don't understand'. Twenty years on I am happy to have discovered the falsehood of that declaration. Derek Milne's text provides a refreshingly clear, informative and stimulating account of the possible contribution which his discipline might make to mine; and I am grateful for it. He does not invite us to become psychologists, but offers, unconditionally, an opportunity to strengthen the foundations of our house. Psychology has served psychiatric medicine well over the last one hundred years, along with support from biology, anthropology, ethology and sociology. Mental health nursing can reap the same benefits without fear that it is, somehow, selling its birthright.

This book places an important item on the agenda of mental health nursing. Nurses need to refine their awareness of the 'patient' if they are to advance their awareness of themselves. Although this is rarely made explicit, psychology appears, to me at least, to be a profession which has little time for introspection. The 'good' psychologist is someone who loses him or herself in knowledge and understanding of others. Through such 'loss' may come 'self-discovery'. The author does not pretend to know all the answers, but is not so foolish as to pretend that some of his uncertainties have not been clarified. He is wise enough, also, to acknowledge some of the mysteries which remain. All in all, this is a book which encourages a critical appreciation of what we 'know', in an effort to extend that knowledge.

This is a book which will stimulate thought, discussion, reflection and further academic research. It is a book which, more importantly, will trigger *action*. The revolution, which people with mental health problems need, must be an academic one: born of philosophy, research and the most considerate of actions. The revolution also demands even better collaboration between professionals and disciplines. This book shows how the knowledge of one discipline can become the practice base of another; and how such practices can, in turn, re-shape the theories which gave them birth. This is no dream scenario. The text is replete with examples of the 'art of the possible': through considera-tion − understanding; through sharing of knowledge − meaningful collaboration; through successful co-operation − effective industry. The goal of successful care (or industry) should provide us with more food for consideration, starting the cycle once more.

I believe that Dr Milne is committed to these ideals, which are not so much lofty as obvious criteria for a humane service to distressed persons. People who require the assistance of mental health nurses would be reassured to know that those charged with their care were being 'shaped' in this admirable fashion. No longer will 'pop psychology' provide an adequate support for those aiming to provide effective, compassionate care. Caring is a serious business; preparation of this order is essential. I have learned many new things from reading this text; I also have recalled much that I had forgotten. I am thankful to the author for his service. I am confident that my colleagues will share my feelings. I am almost certain that people-in-care will feel that their psyches are now in more capable hands.

Phil Barker
Clinical Nurse Consultant
Mental Health Unit
Tayside Health Board
and
Honorary Lecturer
Department of Psychiatry
University of Dundee

Acknowledgements

I am grateful to Cassy Spearing of BPS Books for the invitation to write this book and for all her subsequent support, sustained on her departure by Susan Pacitti. Significant assistance has also been provided by the following mental health nurses, who kindly described a 'case study' from their work for inclusion in the book (number in brackets gives the relevant chapter): Diane Childs (3), Eugene Moynihan (3, 6, 10), Chris Stevenson (4), Dave Reed (5), Judith Elliott (7), Tony Railton (8), Alan Smith and John Wilson (9), and Steve Canham, Bev Hanson and Alan White (10). Helpful comments on drafts were kindly provided by Phil Barker, Geoff Bourne, Dave Bowler, Nick Holdsworth, Richard Marshall, Judy Milne, Dave Müller, Dave Rhodes, Cassy Spearing and Tony Ward. Photographs were taken by Keith Mills and Rob Jordan, and the figures were drawn by Steve Conway. General support and encouragement were provided by my colleagues in the Northumberland District Psychology Service, especially Roger Paxton and Sheila Sharkey. Butterworth Scientific Ltd gave permission to reproduce *Figure 5.1* from West, J. and Spinks, P. (1988) *Clinical Psychology in Action*, London: Wright. Finally a major thank you is due to Barbara Kirkup for her tireless secretarial support. I hope that the book provides them all with some recompense for their help.

Preface

I remember all too clearly my first attempt to try and introduce mental health nurses to the relevance of psychology. After an hour's lecture on the role of the clinical psychologist, a perplexed student piped up with the question 'yes, but what is clinical psychology?' I believe that this book provides a much more straightforward and appropriate answer than that first feeble effort.

Project 2000, the new preparation for nursing practice in the UK, emerged during the late 1980s, a decade after that disastrous lecture. It represented a watershed in the development of education and training in nursing, recognising the need for a fresh and flexible approach to health care needs. This book is a clinical psychologist's response to Project 2000, intended to prepare new students for mental health nursing. In particular, the book uses a problem-solving framework to provide a basis for the nurse of the future, the 'knowledgeable doer' of Project 2000.

I am enthusiastic about this development and very much hope that the book achieves its main aim of offering mental health nurses useful strategies, concepts and methods from a psychological perspective. There is little doubt in my mind that the combination of nursing and psychology has the potential to make the new approach an impressive reality. Certainly the book offers the reader many examples, as well as many new opportunities to integrate the two.

The book is structured to reflect a problem-solving approach to mental health nursing. The recurring theme is that the major challenges of nursing can be reduced to manageable, and even inviting, steps by such a systematic strategy. Indeed, it holds out the prospect of positive developments in the way that nursing is conducted. The four main elements of a problem-solving approach (as in the nursing process) form the basis of the book, namely assessment, planning, implementation and evaluation. Two chapters are devoted to each of these headings, preceded by two introductory chapters and concluded with a synthesis.

Each of the central chapters is supplemented by case study material and exercises. These are intended to flesh out the material and to provide an opportunity for readers to test some of it out for themselves. The chapters end with some key questions and suggestions for further reading, to further encourage involvement in the material. The text is a blend of theory, research and practical guidelines, intended to provide some basic guidance but more importantly to foster an educated, problem-solving approach. The case studies draw on the work of mental health nurses working in the Mental Health Unit of the Northumberland Health Authority, based at St George's Hospital, Morpeth. They show that theory and research can be integrated into nursing practice to produce the flexible and knowledgeable 'doer' of the 1990s.

Derek Milne, Morpeth

SECTION ONE
Setting the scene

1 Introduction

Mental health nursing strode vigorously into the health care world of the 1990s and is developing a coherent and 'transformed' identity (Cawley, 1990). In particular, the advent of the 'nursing process' has given nurses the opportunity to develop a systematically planned and evaluated approach to work. This problem-solving approach is based on the dimensions of assessment, planning, implementation and evaluation (Ward, 1985). These elements are present in a wide range of problem-solving activities outside the field of nursing, since they provide a systematic approach to all kinds of challenges. Walton (1986) notes comparable approaches in education, management, research and other caring occupations. She concluded that the nursing process has helped the profession to move away from the old cliché that doctors are in the *curing* business, while nurses are in the *caring* business. In addition, 'caring' has metamorphosed from a somewhat passive and pejorative term to one that is recognised as broad and central to nursing (McFarlane, 1976). By comparison, the nursing process has negative connotations for many nurses, being associated with endless paperwork. To avoid these negative associations the phrase 'problem-solving approach' is preferred in this book.

Although nursing has progressed, I would emphasise with Cormack (1983) a fundamental difference between statements concerning the way in which nursing should be developing ('prescriptions') and systematic descriptions of what has actually been achieved. In his view, 'psychiatric nurses are still largely concerned with supporting the treatment prescribed by medical staff' (p24). A rather different conclusion emerges in this book although, like Cormack, I believe that the prescriptions are well in advance of the changes in nursing practice.

The aims of this book

Given that the nursing process as a problem-solving strategy can be applied to diverse challenges, I propose to use it to structure this book, since in writing it I face the challenge of highlighting the psychology of most relevance to nursing. It is assumed that nurses have always made use of some of the ideas and methods of psychology, an inevitable consequence of being one group of people working to help another. Much in psychology is 'common sense', and sensible psychological care can emerge from using the resources of this knowledge base in nursing practice. However, as Niven and Robinson (1993) have suggested, this is by no means a straightforward process, and faulty care practices can, and do, emerge.

This book sets out to recognise the important psychological theories in the context of psychiatric nursing activities. It reviews a wide range of psychological theory, research and practice, principally from the literature of clinical psychology. Appropriate links are made to the general psychological literature, largely via the introductory text to this series (Niven and Robinson, 1993). For instance, in dealing with the first stage of the nursing process – assessment – I consider the role of the *therapeutic alliance*, that is, the working relationship between therapist and client, alongside the inevitable differences in the client's and therapist's perceptions of 'the problem'.

The book also recommends further refinements and developments in mental health nursing, resulting in a definite 'handbook' tone to some chapters. This reflects my own perception of problem solving, which is that to make progress, knowledge should be systematically applied in practical situations. My own inspiration is drawn from service evaluation and the scientist-practitioner approach to one's work (Milne, 1987): this is similar to the idea of a 'knowledgeable practitioner' (UKCC, 1987). Both of these approaches involve building on existing ideas from the clinic and from research, by evaluating their application in local services: in good practice we take what is relevant from the work of others and apply it carefully to our own. The ideas and the practice are research-based. The over-riding aim of this book, therefore, is to help mental health nurses of all grades, but especially students undertaking the Mental Health Branch of Project 2000 to take, and apply, the research-based approach from clinical psychology. I believe that it affords another significant step forward in nursing and in the quality of care that nurses provide.

The structure of the book

Following this introductory chapter, the book deals with the 'context' of mental health nursing. Four types of context are discussed. The 'professional' context considers roles, while the 'team' context addresses issues for the nurse in multi-disciplinary working. These levels of activity are set in the wider contexts of the 'community' and the wider 'environment'. This chapter makes explicit the place that our work world plays in shaping what we do.

The next eight chapters follow the headings of the nursing process. There are two chapters on each of the stages of 'assessment', 'planning', 'implementation' and 'evaluation'. In each chapter, theory and practice are blended together, exemplified by the inclusion of case studies and exercises. They are intended to illustrate the relevance of some psychological ideas and methods in a large and typical psychiatric hospital, as well as in the adjoining community services. The exercises are scattered throughout the text and are intended to encourage you to test out psychologically relevant material, such as observing and recording different forms of psychotherapy. As a result of undertaking these exercises you should also be helped to develop your understanding of some key issues. The eleventh and final chapter pulls together the book's themes and offers some recommendations for practice.

The scope of the book

Mental health nursing is a vast topic, subsuming whole disciplines such as psychology, medicine and sociology. Each of these is, in turn, a field with enormous amounts of potentially relevant material. In writing this book I am keenly aware of the difficulty in doing justice to psychology, and although I have done my best to cover the main ideas and applications in this field, I realise that ultimately this is only a sample.

This difficulty reminds me of a piece of Zen wisdom: 'we must live within the ambiguity of partial freedom, partial power and partial knowledge' (Kopp, 1973). I have more difficulty accepting another Zen truth, namely that 'progress is an illusion' (ibid). In the decade since Altschul's (1981) critique, there is a definite impression that in mental health nursing strides have been taken; more may follow. I hope that this book assists the transition and helps to prove that the progress being made in mental health nursing is not illusory.

Explanatory models in mental health nursing

A model is a simplified representation of reality, which helps us to make sense of, and respond to complex matters. By importing ideas from one sphere (such as engineering) and applying them to another (such as nursing), models can be useful in organising and directing our thinking and action. They are not 'real' or 'true', but rather they provide some insight, similar to the function of metaphors in language (for example, 'my head is swimming') in that they help us to understand something, even though we know they are not strictly true (Warr, 1980).

Models may take the form of concrete representations, for example, a model aeroplane, or conceptual representations, such as a particular philosophy of care, or a mathematical formula. Concrete models resemble the real object in central respects – real and model aeroplanes both have the same parts in the same proportions – but differ in others, such as size and ability to fly. Conceptual models, by contrast, are only assumed to have some link to the concept of the subject under study, rather than be an actual representation. If they appear to have some relevance, and to afford a better way of understanding or acting in relation to the object of interest, they may be taken from any sphere.

Nursing models

Nurses have always used models; Hayward's (1986) consideration of models noted that nurses inevitably have a perspective on the nature of their work and how it should be done. For example, Florence Nightingale had a model in which the powers of nature were paramount. She said that nursing 'ought to signify the proper use of fresh air, light, warmth, cleanliness, quiet and the proper selection of and administration of diet' (cited in McFarlane, 1976, pp 195–6). Other nurses have adopted a medical model in which nature is replaced by the technology of EEGs and psychotropic medication.

Latterly, however, the implicit has become much more explicit, as nurses have turned their attention to the nature and utility of their models. To illustrate, consider Roper *et al.*'s (1980) model of nursing which focuses on 12 'activities of living', including 'communicating', 'maintaining a safe environment' and 'breathing'. Each activity has many dimensions – for instance 'communicating' includes verbal and non-verbal forms. The activities of living are also seen as interrelated, for example breathing and communicating. In addition, Roper *et al.* (1980) describe three further dimensions: life-span or development; dependence/independence; and circumstances (such as environmental factors or physical handicaps), which overlap with, and influence, the 12 activities of living. Roper *et al.*'s (1980) model explains individual differences by considering such aspects as how, where and why the activities of living occur. A hierarchy of needs is used to make sense of the way in which these are prioritised. It is noted that a change in circumstances, such as a serious illness, can dramatically alter needs and priorities.

Roper *et al.*'s model is one of many proposed by nurses as ways of thinking about their work. Another popular one is Roy's (1980) 'adaptation' model, which is based on eight assumptions about people. Central to these is the notion that we constantly interact with our environment, adapting to it by means of our biological, psychological and social 'models'. According to Roy's model, the goal of nursing is to promote the client's adaptation, in terms of physiological needs, self-concept, role functioning and social relations. As Riehl and Roy (1980) point out, these and other models of nursing share more similarities than differences. On the basis of this, they offer a 'unified nursing model' which has at its heart a complex being interacting with the environment. The nurse's role is to maintain the client's health 'system', while helping the client to fulfil potential.

Psychological models

Both of the nursing models outlined here have strong psychological elements, but Roy's (1980) seems to have a far greater psychological emphasis: the notion of adaptation is one that has a long and distinguished history in psychology. Several authors have been associated with its development into what is now generally referred to as a 'coping model' (for example, Moos, 1976; Lazarus and Folkman, 1984). Essentially, this model consists of the elements of 'stress' (events which tax our coping repertoire), 'coping' (ways of coping, including personal coping strategies and social support), and 'strain' (the effect of stress with which we are unable to cope). This coping model is set out in Chapter 5 (see *Figure 5.2*). A person's style of coping is part of his or her personality, in that it is their characteristic way of responding to events. It will be shaped in part by biology and partly by environment. The coping model is sufficiently broad in scope to encompass more specific psychological models, such as the intrapsychic one associated with Freud.

In addition to the coping model, to which Freud's work contributed, there are two other major psychological models: the phenomenological model and the behavioural model. *Table 1.1* sets these out in comparison to the biophysical or 'medical' model, according to seven criteria. The critieria include the information (or data) which the model regards as important and the ways in which each model construes problems (the 'definition of pathology'). These criteria help to underline the powerful effect a model has on the way a problem is perceived. To illustrate, in the biophysical model a problem is explained in terms of disease, and the data of interest come from assessments of anatomy and physiology, as inspired by key figures such as Kraeplin. The main concepts used to make sense of disease include genes, the individual's constitution and any observed physical defects. Pathology is defined in terms of failures in these areas and understood to be caused by heredity or environment. Finally, the problem ('pathology') is described in terms of such 'disease' categories as 'anxiety' or 'schizophrenia'. In contrast, the second column in *Table 1.1* outlines the 'intrapsychic' model, which differs markedly in its explanation, data gathering and ideas on the problem. As a result of adopting one of these models, the practitioner will focus on distinctive ways of assessing, understanding and helping clients.

These models drawn from clinical psychology say more about mental health than prevalent nursing ones such as those of Roy and Roper, and

Table 1.1 *The biophysical (or 'medical') model in relation to three dominant ones from clinical psychology (after Eisdorfer et al. 1981)*

	Biophysical	Intrapsychic	Phenomeno-logical	Behavioural
Basic model	Disease	Adaptation	Dissonance	Learning
Data	Heredity; anatomy; physiology etc.	Free association; memories; dreams	Self-reports of conscious attitudes and feelings	Overt behaviour, observed and recorded objectively
Major theorists	Sheldon, Kraeplin	Freud, Jung	Rogers	Skinner, Pavlov
Major concepts	Genes; constitution; defects	Instinct; ego; unconscious	Self; self-regard	Conditioning; reinforcement; generalization
Definition of pathology	Biological (dysfunction; pathology)	Unresolved conflicts; repressed anxieties	Self-discomfort	Maladaptive behaviour
Cause of pathology	Hereditary; constitution	Instincts; deprivation; childhood anxiety	Denied self-actualization	Deficient or maladaptive learning
Types of pathology	Psychiatric categories (e.g. 'schizo-phrenia')	Symptom disorders; character patterns	Impoverish-ment; disorganization	Specific behavioural excesses or deflects

are of great interest to mental health nurses. Also, being longer-standing, these models are buttressed by a large amount of research and theory, so that even if as a nurse you would not align yourself with any of them, they do provide sophisticated models of models. For these reasons, the dominant models in clinical psychology will be introduced throughout the text, as will a few less common ones, such as the family 'systems' model, when these serve to better illustrate a point.

The choice of terms

Bentall *et al.* (1988) addressed one outstanding example of the perennial problem of labelling, that of 'schizophrenia'. Their argument is that the term 'schizophrenia' should be abandoned, as it has proved unhelpful in thinking about, researching or treating those who have been so labelled. Their argument is the latest in a long series of critiques against the use of the term. Notable amongst the earlier antagonists are Szasz (1961) and Laing (1967), who argued that 'schizophrenia' could not be regarded as an illness since no biological explanation had been found and that, rather, the phenomenon was a healing, psychedelic reaction to family persecution.

In reply to Bentall *et al.* (1988), Wing (1988) agreed that arguments about diagnostic categories in general had a long history. At one extreme, he noted, it was argued that states of madness dissolve into each other like clouds in the sky. At the other extreme, proponents argued that clouds can usefully be classified. He suggested that we cannot help categorising things, and that generally this has stood us in good stead. Not least, the terms have remained in use. However, Wing noted the need, in the human sciences particularly, to move from categories to dimensions. That is, in order to provide accurate terms, we need to recognise that phenomena such as 'schizophrenia' are not either present or absent. Rather, there is a continuity between 'normal' and 'abnormal' states. The terms we use to refer to people should therefore recognise the extent to which they experience or exhibit symptoms such as auditory hallucinations.

Unfortunately, this logical requirement flies in the face of the demands of everyday communication, which requires the shortest possible terms so as to limit what people have to say to refer to things. For this reason there is a tendency to use such terms as 'schizophrenia', 'anxiety' and 'depression', even though it is often clearly recognised that these are very loose ways of describing abnormalities in the way people think, feel or behave. In addition, it is acknowledged that such terms or 'labels' can carry unpleasant or undesirable connotations. For instance, the label 'mentally ill' implies certain things about a person's level of responsibility or dependency. Similarly, 'psychiatric hospital' connotes a place where 'madness', an irreversible and inexplicable illness, is treated over long periods of time in the mysterious circumstances of the 'place on the hill'. Altschul (1981) believes that nurses have learnt that labelling tends to result in behaviour to match:

> Once we call sufferers 'patients' they soon adopt a 'sick role'
> every bit as passive as the former inmate role. The sick role confers
> on the 'patient' the right to self-indulgence, the right to
> expect medical care and treatment. It absolves him to a large
> extent of responsibility for his behaviour, but it deprives
> him of the power to make decisions about his own care, to be
> involved in determining his own life pattern (p96).

Similar points are made in relation to the terms 'hospital' and 'nurse'.

There are, therefore, good reasons for changing our use of psychiatric terms, but alongside these is a conflicting communication need to use short and common terms. Attempts to resolve this dilemma have taken several forms, including adding 'person' to terms to emphasise the client's individuality and essential humanity, as in the term 'elderly person' instead of 'geriatric'. Other tactics include referring to people as 'service users' or 'clients'. Service settings become 'homes', or cease to have such stigmatised labels altogether and merge with the terms used for neighbouring abodes – that is, becoming just a number in a street. Similarly, services become 'normalised' and recede anonymously into the language used for other community provisions, so that a service for those with AIDS and HIV infection becomes known as the 'community service'.

A compromise on terms

It can be seen that using such terms attaches less stigma and affords easier communication, but this may be at the cost of reduced accuracy – the local church may also provide a 'community service'. However, this seems to be the best available solution, and is particularly acceptable when those who use such key terms as 'client' are aware of its more precise meaning. In this book, I therefore wish to follow the use of common terms where no better one exists. Thus I will use the main diagnostic categories, such as 'depression' and 'anxiety', and the most popular expressions for service providers and users, such as 'staff' or 'professionals', and 'clients' or 'residents'. I will also use the terms 'problems' and 'difficulties', even though I will explicitly redefine these in terms of a client's 'needs' and 'challenges' later in the book. All these terms are used because they ease communication. Difficulties over stigma and accuracy remain, but these will be addressed throughout the text. The tone will, I hope, indicate that 'clients' are seen in the same light as everyone else, while the general model used exemplifies this by regarding everyone as having to cope with stress and strain. Equally, I will improve the accuracy of terms like 'anxiety' by defining them in context, for example by indicating how a questionnaire sets about measuring the phenomenon. However, I find some terms too vague, unsavoury or misleading to use. These include 'mental illness', 'psychosis' and 'neurosis', and related terms such as 'neurotics'. If such terms are meaningful or useful to the reader, I hope that they will find some way of relating them to the text. Definitions of these terms are to be found in books on psychiatry, such as that by Slater and Roth (1969).

By way of outline, the two main forms of 'mental illness', or 'disorder', are the 'psychoses' and 'neuroses'. A *psychosis* includes

Table 1.2 *A psychological classification of the main problem areas in the 'neurotic' category of adult mental health*

Problem category	Representative difficulties	Illustrations
1. Stress and anxiety	Phobias, obsessional – compulsive disorders	Fear of crowded places; handwashing rituals to remove perceived contamination
2. Interpersonal	Sexual and marital dysfunction	Premature ejaculation; loss of sexual pleasure; communication difficulties
3. Habit disorder	Eating disorders (anorexia, bulimia); dependencies (alcohol, drugs)	Body image distortion; binging and purging re: food, alcohol abuse
4. Depression	Over-arousal; helpless-ness; hopelessness	Hyperactivity; loss of interest; sleep disturbance
5. Educational and occupational	Problems in studying or working	Concentration; poor relationships; mood disturbance
6. Physical health	Poor adjustment to physical illness	Pain; compliance with treatment; delayed healing response
7. Neuropsychological	Cognitive impairment	Problems with various brain activities (e.g. remembering, reasoning, planning)

characteristic disturbances to thought, perception, affect, relationship to the external world and psychomotor behaviour. For example, in 'schizophrenia', the client may experience hallucinations, bizarre delusions and a marked loss of interest in everything. A *neurosis* is characterised by symptoms of anxiety and avoidance behaviour, and unrealistic or excessive anxiety and worry about life circumstances are a central feature. There are numerous disease entities within each of these two categories. For example, the psychoses include 'schizophrenia' and 'delusional disorder'. Depression (and other mood disorders) may be represented as psychotic *or* neurotic, depending on such factors as its severity and duration. The neuroses include 'panic disorder', 'generalised anxiety disorder', 'phobias' and 'obsessive-compulsive disorder' (DSM III R, 1987).

As the orientation of this book is psychological, I will use descriptive categories and terms where appropriate rather than psychiatric terminology. *Table 2.1* sets out the main 'neurotic' categories, following Robson *et al.* (1984). 'Psychotic' problems will generally be discussed in terms of the specific difficulties that present, as in suicidal behaviour or loss of social skills. In Chapters 7 and 8 I will be detailing the kinds of support and therapy that are helpful for both problem categories.

As the focus of the book is on adult mental health, I will not address the sometimes closely related problems which occur with children and with adults who have a learning disability (mental handicap). These groups are the focus of the companion texts in this series.

Summary

This book adopts the four main nursing process elements in order to recognise, review and recommend an expanded link between mental health nursing and psychology. Case studies will illustrate these links, while exercises will help you try out relevant ideas. The book aims to assist mental health nurses to take another stride towards improved care practices. It does so by taking evidence from psychological research, developing applications and encouraging their adoption in a cautious, research-minded approach to one's work.

One way in which psychology can contribute to nursing is by suggesting potentially useful models. Three popular ones are outlined and will appear throughout the text. Psychology can also help you to understand the importance of the language that is used in nursing. Many terms merely serve to label the clients we seek to help, thus exaggerating their difficulties. The importance of reaching a balance between the power of labels such as 'depression' to describe something in a way that eases the task of communication, and conversely their power to encourage faulty ideas and expectations of the bearer of the label, is stressed.

References

Altschul, A. T. (1981). Issues in Psychiatric Nursing. In L. Hockey (Ed.). *Recent Advances in Nursing 1: Current Issues in Nursing*. Edinburgh: Churchill-Livingstone.

Bentall, R. P., Jackson, H. F. and Pilgrim, D. (1988). Abandoning the concept of 'schizophrenia': Some implications of validity arguments for psychological research into psychotic phenomena. *British Journal of Clinical Psychology, 27*, 303–324.

Cawley, R. H. (1990). Educating the psychiatrist of the 21st Century. *British Journal of Psychiatry, 157,* 174–181.

Cormack, D. F. S. (1983). *Psychiatric Nursing Described.* Edinburgh: Churchill-Livingstone.

Diagnostic & Statistical Manual of Mental Disorders (DSM III R, 1987). 3rd edn., revised. Washington: American Psychiatric Association.

Eisdorfer, C., Cohan, D., Kleinman, A. and Maxim, P. (1981). *Models for Clinical Psychopathology.* New York: SP Medical and Scientific Books.

Hayward, J. (Ed; 1986). *Report of the Nursing Process Education Working Group.* London University: Nursing Research Unit. (Report No. 5).

Kopp, S. (1973). *If you meet the Buddha on the road, kill him.* London: Sheldon Press.

Laing, R. D. (1967). *The Politics of Experience.* London: Penguin.

Lazarus, R. S. and Folkman, S. (1984). *Stress, Appraisal and Coping.* New York: Springer.

McFarlane, J. K. (1976). A charter for caring. *Journal of Advanced Nursing, 1,* 187–196.

Milne, D. L. (1987). *Evaluating Mental Health Practice: Methods and Applications.* London: Routledge.

Moos, R. H. (Ed; 1976). *Human Adaptation: Coping with Life Crises.* Lexington, Mass.: D. C. Heath and Co.

Niven, N. and Robinson, J. (1993). *The Psychology of Nursing Care: A foundation text.* Leicester: BPS Books (The British Psychological Society) and London: Macmillan.

Riehl, P, and Roy, C. (1980). *Conceptual Models for Nursing Practice.* (2nd edn.) Norwalk: Appleton-Century-Crofts.

Robson, M. H., France, R. and Bland, M. (1984). Clinical Psychologist in Primary Care: Controlled Clinical and Economic Evaluation. *British Medical Journal, 288,* 1805–1808.

Roper, N., Logan, W. W. and Tierney, A. J. (1980). *The Elements of Nursing.* Edinburgh: Churchill-Livingstone.

Roy, C. (1980). The Roy adaptation model. In: J. P. Riehl and C. Roy *Conceptual Models for Nursing Practice.* Norwalk: Appleton-Century-Crofts.

Slater, E. and Roth, M. (1969). *Clinical Psychiatry* 3rd edn. London: Balliere Tindall and Cassell.

Szasz, T. S. (1961). *The Myth of Mental Illness.* New York: Harper and Row.

United Kingdom Central Council (UKCC) (1987). *Project 2000: the final proposals* (Project Paper 9). London, UKCC, 23 Portland Place, London W1N 3AF.

Walton, I. (1986). *The Nursing Process in Perspective: A Literature Review.* York: University Department of Social Policy and Social Work.

Ward, M. F. (1985). *The Nursing Process in Psychiatry.* Edinburgh: Churchill-Livingstone.

Warr, P. B. (1980). An introduction to models in psychological research. In A. J. Chapman and D. M. Jones (Eds) *Models of Man.* Leicester: BPS Books (The British Psychological Society).

Wing, J. K. (1988). Abandoning what? *British Journal of Clinical Psychology, 27,* 325–328.

Further reading

Buss, D. M. (1990). Toward a biologically informed psychology of personality. *Journal of Personality, 58,* 1–16.
   Buss's is one of the papers from the special issue of the *Journal of Personality.*

He describes nine ways in which biological approaches can inform our understanding of the way that people characteristically behave. These include describing and explaining behaviour, identifying individual differences, and providing insights into how personality develops.

Chapman, A. J. and Jones, D. M. (Eds, 1980). *Models of Man*. Leicester: BPS Books (The British Psychological Society).
Based on a conference held in Cardiff, this book brings together contributions from leading psychologists on the nature of models.

Hall, J. N. (1990). Towards a psychology of caring. *British Journal of Clinical Psychology*, *29*, 129–144.
'Caring' has re-emerged as a term describing valued and varied work. In this scholarly review, John Hall considers such features as the philosophies of care reflected by different forms of caring and the emotions associated with caring.

Journal of Personality (1990), 58:1.
A special issue of this journal was dedicated to the role played by biology in personality. It includes articles considering the place of genetics, physiology, adaptation and evolution, as well as several which focus on the interaction between biology and environment. This link helps to explain some of the ways in which clients cope with stressors, as well as why they sometimes misperceive stressful events.

Wolfensberger, W. (1972). *The Principle of Normalisation in Human Services*. Toronto: National Institute on Mental Retardation.
Wolfensberger's work, to promote the principle of socially valued roles, has been a major influence in the field of learning disabilities. Like Tajfel's book, this one is concerned with the effects of labels and groupings.

Tajfel, H. (1981). *Human groups and social categories*. Cambridge: University Press.
Tajfel is a social psychologist who has developed 'social identity theory'. This holds that a person's identity, self-concept and self-esteem depend at least partly on the social categories (groups) to which they belong and hence is relevant to the earlier discussion on the terms used.

2 *The context of mental health nursing*

One of the truisms of psychology is that the things we observe occur in a context: behaviour does not take place in a vacuum. All the models considered in Chapter 1 emphasised the relationship between behaviour and important events going on inside or outside the client. For the psychodynamic model this may consist of unconscious processes such as 'denial', while for the behaviourist the onus is placed on events taking place around the patient, such as social activities. Despite such differences, they both share the view that the individual's behaviour occurs for a reason outside the individual's knowledge or control, and is not simply the result of 'free will'. It follows that behaviour can only be properly understood in the light of those factors known to influence it. The models disagree about the nature of these influences, but not about their existence or importance. These factors are the *context* for everyone's behaviour, whether we are clients, nurses or psychologists. Examples of these different models of therapy are to be found in Chapter 6.

The professional context of mental health nursing

We are all familiar with the broad distinctions between the various professional groups involved in mental health services. We may know that social workers visit a patient's family and take a keen interest in their history, or that psychiatrists tend to focus on diagnosis and medication. We are probably also aware that when examined more closely, these professional groups have considerable areas of overlap (try *Exercise 2.1* as an example). For instance, most disciplines aim to provide some kind of assessment and treatment for psychological complaints. Furthermore, several of these disciplines will use apparently identical methods in order to give this help.

For example, mental health nursing has been defined as work intended to promote mental health through restoration and prevention, based on providing comprehensive and individualised nursing interventions to clients, relatives and others (ENB, 1989). Such general terms are inevitably applicable to other professional groups, so this definition must hinge on what is meant by 'nursing'.

Exercise 2.1: Roles in multidisciplinary teams
Study the following list of activities and decide which one represents which professional group. You should try and identify community psychiatric nursing, social work, psychiatry and clinical psychology. The answers are given at the end of the chapter, after the References (see p. 42).

Group 1	Group 2	Group 3	Group 4
diagnostician	clinician	relapse preventer	diagnostician
planner	staff supporter	assister with employment and accommodation adviser	psycho-therapist
adviser	teacher	supporter	drug treat-ment provider
enabler	supervisor	assister with practical needs (e.g. nutrition)	co-ordinator
counsellor	service planner	agency co-ordinator	physical examiner
social educator	researcher	domiciliary therapy provider	teacher
consultant	evaluator		problem formulator
researcher	innovator		
advocate	manager		
care-giver			

A good illustration of the overlap between disciplines has been the common interest of 'nurse therapists' and psychologists in behaviour therapy. This form of therapy emphasises observable problem behaviours, which are altered by changing the client's environment (for example, through a nurse offering praise to a dependent client who has carried out a behaviour independently, such as using the toilet appropriately). Nurse therapists have emerged because of the tremendous demand for skilled therapists, the gradual extension of the nurse's clinical role, and the development of methods that are relatively readily learned and effective (Barker, 1982). They have undertaken post-basic training for up to 18 months and have then practised behaviour therapy in the same way as clinical psychologists. It is not uncommon now to find a Health Centre with both a psychologist and a nurse therapist, with the general practitioner referring similar patients to both of them. It is also widely acknowledged by psychologists (the original behaviour therapists) that the nurses have a better training in this approach. Given the striking degree of overlap that exists between professionals working in the mental health field, how can we (or our clients) tell them apart? Perhaps as a result of this apparent confusion, attempts have been made to distinguish between professional roles.

An example of role clarification

Community psychiatric nursing (CPN) has been described in terms of the work activities for Group 3 in *Exercise 2.1*. This includes visiting clients at home in order to maintain treatment (for example, giving injections) and serving as a co-ordinator between hospital, community and other health care agencies. However, it is recognised that there is no consensus of opinion on the CPN's role. In order to try and clarify matters, Wooff *et al.* (1988) observed the work of ten CPNs and ten mental health social workers in Salford Health District. Both groups saw similar clients, referred to them largely by general practitioners and psychiatrists. However, CPNs focused on treatment and symptoms approximately twice as often as the social workers, who focused rather on the clients' welfare, daily living, relationships and so on. Analysis of the speech of the CPNs and social workers showed clear differences. For CPNs, 30 per cent of their speech focused on symptoms (physical and psychiatric) and 29 per cent on medication and its administration. In contrast, the social workers spent 47 per cent of their time talking about interpersonal relationships, symptoms, and finances, and only half as much time on symptoms and medication. Indeed, they spent far more time with each client, an average of 25 minutes, compared to 16 minutes given by the CPNs. This perhaps reflected their greater use of counselling and related methods: these methods were used in 77 per cent of client consultations, compared to 22 per cent of the CPNs' client consultations, (all non-schizophrenic clients). In 45 per cent of their cases, the social workers also planned to involve other mental health workers more, compared to 23 per cent for the CPNs. Summing up these findings, Wooff *et al.* (1988) stated that while there were areas of overlap, 'CPNs primarily applied a biological model of care while social workers mainly applied a psychosocial model' (p789).

Two points are worth highlighting at this stage. Firstly, as stressed by Wooff and by Paykel and Griffith (1983), differences between professional groups are essentially desirable, since this provides the broad range of services many clients require, while simultaneously giving the professionals themselves a clear sense of their own identity. The second point is that general statements of work roles are usually misleading: both social workers and CPNs claim to provide forms of therapy and support to their clients, but on closer inspection these turn out to be rather different services.

Defining general aspects of professional roles

Given findings such as these, it becomes necessary to consider how best to distinguish between the different professions. Clearly a major difficulty in describing one's role, and in drawing distinctions between professions, lies in the very general terms that are used. 'Counselling' for instance, covers anything from disciplinary action to a sophisticated form of psychotherapy. A more accurate definition of terms would enable us to say how apparently similar professional activities actually do differ, and demonstrate how members of the same profession differ in their pursuit of the same activities.

In order to consider these points in more detail, let us look at some psychotherapy research which has been undertaken in Sheffield (Shapiro and Firth, 1987). Two basic kinds of psychotherapy were compared, *prescriptive* and *exploratory*. The prescriptive therapy was a combination of cognitive and behavioural therapies, including forms of anxiety management such as relaxation and graded exposure to feared stimuli, and methods of altering the ways in which the client thinks about problems (for example, the therapist challenging irrational beliefs). Exploratory therapy was based on counselling and psycho-dynamic methods, with an emphasis on enhancing the client's 'insight' or self-awareness. This was achieved through the therapeutic relation-ship. (These two forms of therapy are discussed in detail in Chapter 6.) Evaluation of the outcomes of these two forms of psychotherapy indicated that the prescriptive therapy was slightly more effective.

This research shows that the shared term 'therapy' can conceal rather different clinical outcomes. But more interestingly, for our present argument, there was also evidence to show that the two therapies involved different kinds of speech from the therapist, as in the social worker and CPN comparison earlier. A 12-category observation system, called the *Helper Behaviour Rating System*, was used to classify what the therapists said. This covered such items as 'interpretation', 'exploration', 'reflection', 'reassurance', 'disagreement', 'open-question' and 'self-disclosure'. Therapists in the 'exploratory' therapy were found to make more use of 'interpretation', 'exploration' and 'process advisement' (that is, comments on what was going on in the session). In the 'prescriptive' therapy they asked more questions, gave more 'information' and 'general advisement' (that is, instructions on things to do after the session). The remaining categories did not significantly differ between the therapies.

These findings indicate that careful analysis of generally labelled activities, such as 'therapy', can reveal important differences both in what takes place during therapy and in the way this effects the client's wellbeing. This information is potentially useful in distinguishing between the work of the different professionals, because it allows us to give more precise and objective labels to their activities. It also provides a basis for a more systematic and efficient approach to multidisciplinary teamwork, by relating what the different team members do in relation to the needs of different clients. As we learn more and more about the 'best' therapies for different mental health difficulties, so we can more successfully match up therapy, therapist and client. This makes more sense than assuming that all team members and all clients are more or less equivalent, and allocating work on this basis, as sometimes happens. Detailed discussion of case work, joint work and mutual observation are other promising ways of distinguishing amongst the contributions that team members can make.

The team context of mental health nursing

The idea of a team of therapists, drawn from different disciplines but working together as equals, dates back to the mid-1970s. It was intended to supersede the traditional approach in which the consultant psychiatrist made all the important decisions and carried out or prescribed most of the treatments. The multidisciplinary team (MDT) was seen as a way of focusing on clients' needs by a combination of 'key worker' links between therapists and clients, case-centred MDT meetings, and the co-ordination of therapists and other services in relation to the client's needs. The MDT was to become the 'gatekeeper' to the full and now more co-ordinated range of mental health services, developing close working links with key referral agents such as general practitioners.

The team was also to spearhead new patterns of care in the community, integrating this with hospital-based services. One example would be the development of home-based assessment of clients who would otherwise be admitted to hospital, forming the basis of discussion and decision-making in the MDT about the most appropriate form of care. This might be an alternative form of residential accommodation or the provision of more intensive help in the client's home.

Multidisciplinary teams can be defined by a number of features:

- the team consists of a group of professionals such as nurse, social worker, psychiatrist, psychologist, occupational therapist;
- members work in the same geographical 'patch', such as a group of hospital wards or a part of a district;
- the team meets regularly for formal case-centred discussions;
- each professional allocates time to attend MDT meetings and to carry out team decisions.

In addition, the MDT will have an agreed, detailed and written statement of its objectives which should govern how the team works.

This contrasts with the traditional 'ward round', which is a medically dominated review of the client's progress, in that, for example, all team members would be expected to work together flexibly, altering or exhanging some aspects of their roles in order to respond better to the needs of the client. No single team member would be expected to override others by virtue of status or power, but rather decisions would be reached by consensus amongst mutually respectful professionals.

The MDT should be distinguished from the looser working arrangement between professionals termed a 'network'. This refers to a less formal collaboration of different disciplines, services, employers and units on the basis of the occasional individual case which creates difficulties within the routine arrangements. In this sense, an MDT may liaise over the care of an individual with voluntary agencies such as Age Concern or MIND, who may in turn link up with informal support providers, such as the client's family or friends.

Difficulties in multidisciplinary teams

Although MDTs were seen as a promising way in which to organise services, in practice they are prone to a number of difficulties which can significantly diminish their value. Amongst the more frequent are unclear objectives, inefficient working relationships, and confusion over responsibility.

Considering these in turn, MDTs may have poorly defined or even non-existent objectives. The team may then have difficulty obtaining guidance from service managers and others, so that they attempt to define objectives on their own. This can lead to a conflict with the priorities of other services, or to unnecessary tension amongst the team because of different emphases.

Even when objectives are clear and agreed, the team can encounter obstacles in its working relationships. Classic examples include role disputes over who is the team 'expert' on a particular therapy; who sees which kinds of clients; and who is the team leader. These can severely undermine the team's efficiency by misdirecting energy and underutilising skills.

These difficulties are not always present, of course, nor are they insuperable. Poorly defined objectives can be a useful challenge to a team, giving it the opportunity to work together to clarify the client needs it is addressing. Related tasks include establishing an identity and way of working together, generating a policy statement, and finding out about relevant resources. All of these will help the team generate a detailed statement of its objectives, which can then be put forward to service managers for approval. Likely benefits of this joint effort are that objectives will be understood, accepted, and related to local circumstances. In turn, this promotes the motivation of team members.

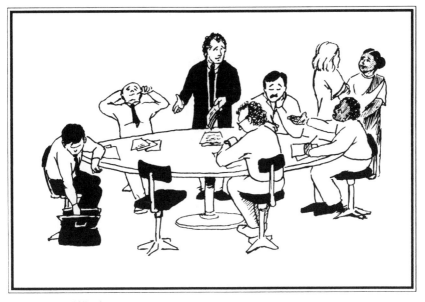

A team in difficulty

Turning to relationships within the MDT teams, difficulties such as accountability, role conflict and leadership can also be resolved. Everyone in the health services has a manager to whom they are accountable. As this person will rarely be a member of the same multidisciplinary team as their junior colleague, some matters will need to be discussed outwith the team. Examples include departmental policies regarding the type of work to be undertaken and the amount of autonomy normally permitted. Tensions created by this dual accountability to the manager and to the multidisciplinary team, can be eased by team members sharing experiences, thus improving mutual understanding and expectations.

Role conflict is a growing difficulty. As already discussed, more and more professional groups are laying claim to more and more of what was formerly only one profession's area of expertise. Within each profession, differences in therapeutic orientation, experience, training and so forth will blur the distinctions still further. This can create considerable tension amongst the team; we will consider this again later. Leadership conflicts are part and parcel of such things as the struggle for power, the danger of losing influence or status, and the resentment of authority figures. But there are usually a number of tasks that need leaders, and it is useful to share these amongst the team according to respective skills and interests. Tasks include ensuring the effective functioning of meetings, representing the team, liaising with other teams, teaching, researching and evaluating. Such a sharing of leadership functions can make the best use of the individual team member's talents, balancing out much of the power and thus paving the way for more commitment and mutual support.

An issue closely related to that of leadership is responsibility. Traditionally the consultant psychiatrist has assumed leadership of other professionals, often on the basis of being the 'responsible medical officer'. However, there does not appear to be any legal basis for this claim; rather, every member of a service (or an MDT) has a 'duty of care' towards their clients requiring them to take 'reasonable care in all circumstances' (British Psychological Society, 1986). All professionals are expected to recognise and stay within the limits of their training and competence. In the UK, there is the *Tort of Negligence*, which makes each professional responsible for his or her own actions. It follows, therefore, that no professional, whether consultant psychiatrist or anyone else, can be held legally responsible for another professional's actions, or claim ultimate or overall responsibility.

This is not to argue that 'medical responsibility' does not exist, but rather to suggest that this is essentially similar to 'nursing responsibility', 'social worker responsibility', and so on; namely, they are all required to work within certain legal, employment and professional boundaries. There is, therefore, no right or requirement for any professional to assume 'leadership' or 'responsibility' over other professionals, but in practice it is often useful for one professional to take 'prime responsibility' for a particular client. This means that the professional acts as co-ordinator for the team's efforts in relation to this client, perhaps undertaking the majority of the assessment and therapy with them, and carrying out other responsibilities, such as monitoring progress and involving other professionals as appropriate. Typically a key worker would assume prime responsibility, but it is crucial that all team members know who has assumed what responsibilities and then work together as effectively as possible for the good of the client.

Of course, we all know that teams don't necessarily function as they should: disputes over responsibilities, and rivalry over roles and expertise are amongst the more common difficulties. What has psychology got to say about this difference between theory and practice in teamwork? In essence, it is the 'motivational' dimension which provides most insight into the difference. That is, people basically know what to do, and generally have the ability to do it. What is missing is the *will* to act and to turn principles into realities.

The motivation to work well within a team is related to many of the things already mentioned, such as professional identity and responsibility. These can be (and frequently are) challenged in team work. In a paper called *Blood and Gore*, Richard Marshall (1989) considered the nature of conflicts from a Freudian perspective. He described the way in which behaviours within teams can operate as a defence against anxieties which are aroused when working closely with clients. In

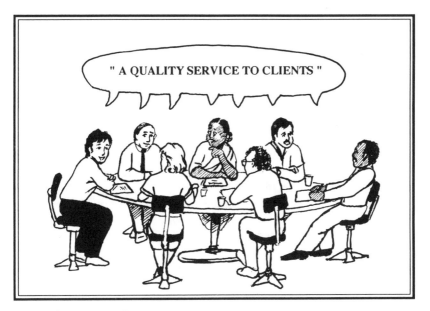

A team in agreement

general, team members will have entered their profession with the expectation that they will be able to make people better. When clients are angry, hostile, withdrawn or reject help, feelings can be aroused which conflict with the team member's perception of him or herself as helpful and caring. In newly formed teams, and in recently qualified professionals, such anxiety will be great as individuals will tend to feel vulnerable and unsure about their role and competence.

In order to cope with these anxieties, team members may distance themselves from the client by depersonalising the client, denying their own feelings and 'splitting' (that is, seeing the client's problems in black and white terms, so that the client is then seen as either entirely 'bad' or entirely 'mad'). This same process may be involved when a team member splits off and projects an aspect of him or herself onto someone else, perhaps denying their capacity for responsible decision making and projecting this onto another, such as a consultant or team leader. If such a process is allowed to develop it can lead to individual team members feeling at times that they have all the authority and skills which others have not, or conversely they may feel inadequate, deskilled and the team scapegoat.

These unconscious coping strategies can have an adverse effect on the functioning of the team. Marshall suggests that we learn who our allies are from a cautious testing of their *actual* support (verbal support is usually unreliable), from being attentive to the different alliances and power struggles within the team, and from developing an understanding of the relationships amongst team members. From this basis, team members can take positive, adaptive steps, and move toward a clear and full use of their own skills, in the knowledge that they have something valuable to contribute.

Factors promoting good teamwork

Other writers (such as West, 1989), have singled out the following four factors as important for successful teamwork:

- *Vision*: having a shared idea of what the team really wants to achieve is the first challenge;
- *Participation*: the more team members are involved in decision-making, the more likely they are to work for the outcomes of those decisions, provided that the risks are acceptable.
- *Focus*: it is necessary to retain sight of the team's aim of providing a top quality service to its clients. There can be a tendency to drift away from this basic goal, while still retaining vision and participation. Regular reappraisal of current practices is a healthy way of maintaining the focus while still improving the service, particularly when based on a constructive monitoring of one another's work.
- *Support*: it is important to seek, and obtain, from managers the resources and encouragement to pursue the team's vision (for example, time to work on ideas, statements of support in meetings, rewards for progress). This enables the team to sustain its focus through to task completion.

West (1989) emphasises that team members may feel powerless in a large organisation such as a psychiatric hospital. For example, a nurse may have great difficulty changing the most basic things, such as the furniture or social routines, in an institution. But West's message is that, by working on the four points mentioned, people can be motivated to work effectively as a team. Llewelyn and Fielding (1983) provide other tips on tackling the conflict which can cripple a team. They highlight the role played by group dynamics, and urge nurse tutors to address this powerful process, which if not halted can lead to different professional groups wasting a great deal of energy defending 'their' expertise or resources, and enforcing loyalty from their own group. The psychology of group behaviour is a relevant backdrop for these team traumas (see Niven and Robinson, 1993).

The 'community context' of mental health nursing

If one accepts the view that it is what professionals actually do that matters, rather than their title or what they say they do, then the next logical step is to consider how other people contribute to the mental health of the community. I refer now to the diverse range of interpersonal help provided by people who do not have an official role in mental health work, such as volunteers. These people provide what has been termed *social support* or *informal psychotherapy*, help which appears to complement the work of the formal therapists. Indeed, there is a fair amount of evidence to suggest that in some respects, these 'para-professionals' may do as good a job as the more highly-trained professionals. Hattie *et al.* (1984) concluded that 'para-professionals are at least as effective, and in many instances more effective, than professional counsellors' (p540). They did, however, qualify this conclusion by surmising that referrals made to the professionals may have been more exacting. However, this, and other reviews of its kind, points to the power of the non-professional in promoting mental health in the community. We would do well to respect and attempt to harness this power.

Perhaps we should begin by analysing what it is that many non-professionals do to help people. Just as we can analyse what formal therapists do, as illustrated in the Sheffield psychotherapy project, so we can analyse the social support provided by non-professionals. Four main activities have been distinguished by a number of researchers:

- *Non-directive support*: listening, expressing esteem, caring and understanding;
- *Tangible assistance*: providing money or materials; helping with tasks;
- *Positive social interaction*: engaging in social interactions for fun or relaxation;
- *Directive guidance*: offering advice, information or instruction.

As we all know from our own experience, all kinds of people provide these forms of help in all kinds of contexts. The most common social support providers are family and friends, but examples of social support can be observed in most interactions involving two or more people.

Exercise 2.2: A social support exercise
In order to clarify these helping activities, you should complete the questionnaire which is at the end of this chapter (see p42). Called the *Inventory of Social Supportive Behavior (ISSB)* Barrera *et al.* 1981), this questionnaire should also show you the range of informal help that you yourself receive. The three types of social support (informational, emotional and practical) are measured by different questionnaire items. Once you have completed and scored the questionnaire, compare notes with a colleague: you will no doubt find that you have different types and sources

of social support. This underlines the individual differences in the help we receive, and emphasises the need to assess each client's informal help rather than making assumptions about its nature, sources or adequacy.

Research on social support

Research surveys suggest that although mental health professionals typically spend most of their working day dealing with psychological problems, there are other jobs which are associated with surprisingly high levels of helping. In a review of such research, Emery Cowen (1982) drew attention to the help provided by hairdressers, lawyers, work supervisors and bartenders. He pointed out that these roles offer inexpensive, accessible and non-stigmatised help, often from people with similar backgrounds and who are therefore particularly well-placed to understand problems and to suggest practical solutions. Maybe because of these factors, it has been found that less than 20 per cent of those who saw themselves as having psychological problems took those problems to mental health professionals.

Cowen (1982) has provided a breakdown of the kinds of personal problems people raise with informal helpers. The most common are problems with children, physical health, relationships, depression,

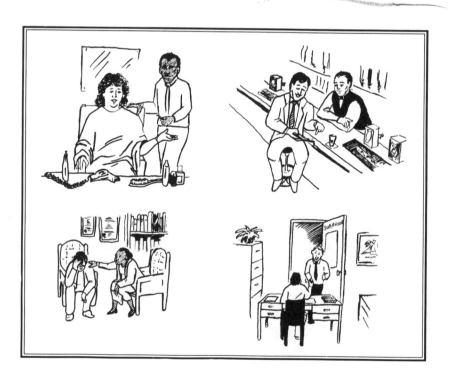

anxiety, work and money. However, the list is 25 items long, and includes more of the less common psychological complaints of guilt, confusion, worthlessness and loneliness. The hairdressers, bartenders, lawyers and supervisors who were studied differed quite noticeably in terms of the sort of problems they were presented with, presumably as a result of their relationship with the 'client' and the nature of the work done.

These helping groups had more in common when it came to their ways of handling personal problems. Most of them offered support and sympathy, tried to be lighthearted, listened and suggested alternatives. Again, however, there was a long list of the strategies used, and again some were strikingly psychological. These included helping the 'client' to clarify feelings, encouraging the 'client' to come up with alternatives and asking questions.

These groups saw their help as a generally enjoyable and important part of their job. However, they had mixed feelings after providing social support, which may reflect their lack of training for the helping role. For example, the hairdressers mostly felt 'gratified', 'sympathetic' and 'supportive', but it was also fairly common for them to feel 'trapped', 'depressed' and 'angry'.

In recognition of the helping role played by hairdressers and others, I have conducted several studies in order to investigate the major questions remaining at the time of Cowen's review (Milne *et al.*, 1992). These included the need for systematic observations of the type of help provided by hairdressers and psychotherapists, and considerations of the impact of the social support role on the helper's own wellbeing and on that of their clients. In the first of these studies, observations were conducted in salons and clinics using the *Helper Behaviour Rating System* (as described in the Sheffield psychotherapy project). The correlation between what stylists and therapists said to their respective clients was non-significant, indicating that they did not speak to their clients in similar ways. Particularly striking, however, were the scores on the *Helper Behaviour Rating System* for 'reassurance', 'advice', 'exploration' and 'interpretation' (all three times more frequent for the therapists). In contrast, stylists gave more information, asked more questions, disagreed more and reflected more of the clients' speech.

A second study provided a workshop for stylists in order to increase their capacity to provide social support. The results suggested that they had benefitted from the 10-hour workshop, achieving higher levels of cognitive and behavioural coping after training, and lower distress. Customer ratings of the stylists' helpfulness remained high throughout the study, showing that the stylists had maintained their social support activities.

In a third study, the impact of the stylists' help on their clients was focused on. This time a workshop was run to develop the ways in which the stylists provided social support. Random samples of clients attending the salon gave significantly higher ratings of the stylists' helpfulness after the workshop, indicating that they were benefiting from better social support.

These three studies show how people with psychological problems may obtain help from their hairdressers, one example of the range of social support providers. Nurses can learn from these examples by analysing the factors which seem to contribute to mental health, and consider how they can facilitate these in hospital or community settings. An emphasis on the relationship between these informal psychotherapists and the mental health professional's clients paves the way towards more natural and potentially more effective health care.

Voluntary help

We have seen how the activities of the different mental health professionals overlap, and that these in turn may merge with the type of help provided by social supporters. Between these two groups lie those voluntary agencies who also provide help to those with psychological problems, but who differ in some respects from the professionals and the social supporters. They usually share the same objectives and source of funding with the professionals (often financed by the public sector – for example, the NHS and Social Services), but will typically differ in having less specialised training and fewer resources. Examples in the UK include Age Concern, The National Schizophrenia Fellowship, The Alzheimers Disease Society, Cruse, and MIND. Their objectives and activities usually distinguish them from social supporters. Although each may at times provide the same kind of accessible help (for example, 'informational support' or reassurance), voluntary agencies stand out in such ways as their use of designated types of help, for example counselling, and designated premises, such as drop-in centres.

Mental health professionals liaise with, and facilitate the work of, voluntary agencies much more commonly than they work with social support systems. They may collaborate over individual clients, perhaps arranging for an elderly person who is being discharged from hospital to have a home help, or providing some support to allow respite to a carer (an Age Concern service). They may also collaborate in developing a service to clients, as the following study involving MIND illustrates.

This study aimed to reduce anxiety, one of the most commonly experienced mental health problems (Milne *et al.*, 1989). Community psychiatric nurses, social workers, psychologists and MIND teamed up in one district to produce a self-help booklet on anxiety management and to organise group therapy for anxious people, based on this booklet. Evaluations suggested this was a clinically effective anxiety management package, and one that was attractive to clients. Groups of ex-clients were taught to train and support other clients, and in so doing took on the role of therapist, thus further blurring the boundaries between formal and informal help. These therapists had undergone successful treatment for their own anxiety before undertaking further training to prepare them to use their own experiences to help others. These groups were all run under the name of local MIND, but were organised by the multidisciplinary team of professionals.

Examples such as these show psychological help to be a complex phenomenon. We can see that there are a range of people who provide help with mental health problems, and that very crudely they can be labelled 'professionals', 'volunteers' and 'social supporters'. The relationships between them are complex, as sometimes they work closely together while at other times they appear to ignore one another's very existence. However, they all face strikingly similar demands from clients, albeit with varying frequency and intensity, and they all share some strategies for dealing with these demands. *Exercise 2.2* is intended to increase your awareness of these points.

In conclusion, the community context of mental health nursing is a powerful determinant of our clients' behaviour. Although challenging and new, it is important for nurses to try to understand and marshal some of their potential allies amongst the ranks of social supporters and volunteers.

The 'environmental' context of mental health nursing

So far, we have considered how the work of a mental health nurse should be understood in the context of the nursing profession, multidisciplinary teamwork and key people in the community. In turn, all of these are part of a more general 'environment', made up of such diverse things as buildings, economics, politics, social class and so forth. To a greater or lesser extent, these are all factors with a bearing on the nurse's work with any client. They impinge directly and indirectly on what we do, whether or not we realise it.

The environmental context is important as it helps us to make sense of behaviour. It stresses that our method of working is not some kind of fixed response, but rather is related to what is going on around us. (This can be contrasted with the view that people, whether clients or therapists, behave as they do because of their 'illness' or some basic biological 'drive'.) This approach suggests that it is an interaction between individual and environment. It has already been suggested that this is the case for more immediate contexts, such as that of teamwork, but let us now consider some of the evidence regarding the importance of these larger environmental factors.

In 1978 a team commissioned to report on mental health to the US President stated that:

> mental health problems cannot be defined only in terms of disabling mental illnesses and identified psychiatric disorders. They must include the damage to mental health associated with unrelenting poverty and unemployment and the institutionalized discrimination that occurs on the basis of race, sex, age and mental and physical handicap. They must also include conditions that involve emotional and psychological distress which do not fit conventional categories of classification or services . . . mental health services cannot adequately respond to the needs of the citizens of this country unless those involved in the planning, organization, and delivery of those services fully recognize the harmful effect that a variety of social, environmental, physical, psychological and biological factors can have on the ability of individuals to function in society, develop a sense of their own worth, and maintain a strong and purposeful self-image (p9; cited in Monahan and Vaux, 1980).

If one accepts this view, what can be done to recognise these environmental factors and use them to the clients' advantage? Let us look at the main factors.

The physical environment: 'settings' as a context for behaviour

It is obvious that all behaviour takes place in the context of a certain time and place, and if we look carefully we would find that these will influence what happens. For instance, in any High Street, the time of five past midnight on the first of January is associated with characteristically happy social scenes. These sorts of behaviours are less likely to occur at other times or in other places (such as a psychiatric hospital's main corridor at the same time). More clinically-relevant examples, such as taking an 'institutionalised' client on an outing, are probably part of everyone's experience. It is not uncommon for the patient to behave in ways not observed in the hospital, the logical inference being that the change of physical environment has influenced his or her behaviour, and usually for the better.

Studies of the relationship between environment and behaviour often start with careful observations, addressing the question of what goes on in the various parts of a hospital or community. A good early example is the work of Willems (1972), who observed what inpatients did in different parts of the hospital. About 90 per cent of all observed behaviour took place in only 4 per cent of the 122 different settings in the hospital. For instance, most behaviour took place in the ward, and consisted of idleness, sleeping, nursing care and hygiene. Other places were highly associated with specific activities, for example the cafeteria with conversation, or the physical recreation room with exercise. Key behaviours, such as client independence, were found to be most common in the cafeteria, followed by the corridors. Paradoxically, this independence was least frequently observed in the places where it would most be expected, namely occupational therapy and recreational therapy, and only noted at an intermediate level in the wards.

There is, therefore, a scientific parallel for the everyday observation that the physical environment shapes behaviour. Other examples are not hard to find:

- the layout of a housing estate affects the selection of friends from amongst one's neighbours, the duration of neighbourly contacts and the number of confrontations about ownership and territory;
- the design of individual properties can reduce domestic crimes such as theft, damage;
- the layout of furniture within a hospital ward lounge can dramatically affect the quality and quantity of social interactions;
- open dormitories, locked nurses' offices, and large, centralised eating areas adversely influence client behaviour;
- high levels of noise disrupt concentration and the performance of complex tasks (especially if it is out of one's control, or is irregular and unpredictable). Noise affects people's tendency to show affiliation, aggression and helping, by increasing the distance at which people feel comfortable with each other;
- the density, or overcrowding of people also appears to interfere with social relationships (for example, disliking others more, perceiving them as less friendly or co-operative), often leading to withdrawal, in the forms of reduced eye contact and less interaction, which in turn leads to helplessness. Perhaps not surprisingly, it follows that factors such as the number of persons sharing a room have been found to be related to psychiatric hospital admissions.

These findings, found with striking consistency by different researchers in different countries, point to the fact that our physical environment plays a major part in influencing client behaviour.

The role of the social environment

Some of these examples anticipate another important part of the environment, namely the people who occupy it. Indeed, a persuasive line of reasoning suggests that client behaviour alters as settings alter, largely because other *people* respond to these changes. This then influences the client's behaviour, rather than the setting itself doing so. To return to our example, the client whose behaviour changes dramatically on an outing may be responding to a dramatic change in the behaviour of the escorting nurse, rather than to any physical aspects of the environment. Even more realistically, all these factors may interact; the coach trip causes the nurse and client to sit together in a more confined space than is normal which, when allied to a more relaxed atmosphere than is normal, leads to more conversation between them. Willems' (1972) research bears out this hypothesis, with more independence and conversation being observed in the hospital cafeteria.

Another tradition, developed by therapeutic communities, is to consider the way in which important social factors such as group cohesion amongst clients, or unspoken disagreements amongst staff, can influence what takes place in a setting. (A therapeutic community is a setting emphasising principles of democratic decision-making and personal accountability, based around regular meetings between staff and residents: Jones, 1968). Behavioural phases or 'cycles' have been identified in many social settings. For example, *harmony → mounting tension → tension peak → resolution*, then round again to *harmony*. There is some evidence suggesting that client behaviour does follow such patterns. For instance, disturbed behaviour on a ward, involving destructive, hostile or dangerous acts, was found to be significantly higher on weekdays than during weekends. This was apparently related to events such as the large meeting of staff and clients prior to the weekend – the *tension peak*.

Another important dimension of any social environment is peer influence. Many difficulties encountered by institutions such as schools and hospitals have been seen in the light of two antagonistic peer groups, the staff and the inmates. A lot of behaviour can be seen as either furthering the aims of the peer group (fellow nurses or fellow clients) or of undermining those of the other, 'out', group.

A fascinating example has been provided by Sanson-Fisher and Jenkins (1978). Their observations in a correctional institution indicated that the inmates (delinquent girls) worked together in a systematic way in order to coerce the staff away from the aims of the institution. In one instance the girls were successful in getting the staff to carry out domestic chores which the institution expected the girls themselves to carry out! They managed this in subtle ways, such as giving positive attention to the staff when they were washing dishes, and the girls were thus able to get away with doing only 2 per cent of such tasks, regarded as 'therapeutic opportunities' by the institution. Sanson-Fisher and Jenkins used these observations to argue for more staff training, focusing on helping staff to discriminate between 'appropriate' and 'inappropriate' client behaviour, and on controlling their own reactions to the girls. Other social factors governing client behaviour include the programme of activities in a ward (including individual therapy), social events (such as Christmas) and the reactions of significant others (for example, family and friends).

The part played by other environmental factors

The list of factors which can influence behaviours, thoughts and feelings is vast, and to cover them all would be beyond the scope of this book. But rather than stopping at physical and social factors in the therapy environment, it may be helpful briefly to indicate the important aspects of some other factors, based on a review by Monahan and Vaux (1980).

Social class has consistently been found to correlate with mental health: the association is that the 'lower' the social class, the higher the frequency of psychological difficulties. This finding goes back to at least 1856, when Jarvis (cited in Monohan and Vaux, 1980) reported that the pauper class in Massachusetts had 64 times as many cases of insanity, proportionately, as the independent class.

The relationship with formal help is reversed, however, with recent studies finding that the 'upper' classes received far more individual psychotherapy, while the 'lower' classes received more physical treatments, such as medication and ECT.

As with any correlational study, these findings beg the question of cause and effect: is lower social class a cause or a consequence of psychological difficulty? As people with some form of difficulty may not rise through the class structure, or may indeed fall through it, there may be a powerful tendency for them to occupy the 'lower' classes. These processes would make psychological difficulty a cause of one's class membership. On the other hand, people in the 'lower' classes may experience more difficulty as a consequence of their living conditions (for example, poverty, poor housing)· this is the *social causation* hypothesis. Research suggests that both processes may be at work.

Unemployment has also been implicated in mental health, as it typically fosters low self-esteem and dissatisfaction with oneself. Suicide occurs more frequently amongst the unemployed and amongst those who drop down a social class. However, the relationship between work and wellbeing is not a simple one, as other factors, such as social support, the general employment situation and the status of one's work skills, may well reduce the impact of unemployment.

A major review of work, unemployment and mental health by Warr (1987) also places these factors within the context of a range of environmental factors. These include the extent to which an individual can establish his or her own goals, have opportunities to use and develop skills, and have a physically secure living environment. The factors were thought to encompass both work and unemployment, and to have the potential to have a significant impact on mental health. In his consideration of mental health, Warr reviewed studies indicating that employment helped clients improve in the areas of anxiety, depression and vigour. He also reviewed some early psycho-dynamic theorising on the role of work, which suggested that for those who were 'neurotically disposed', it served to control inner impulses and punishment fantasies. This was indicated by the so-called 'Sunday neuroses'. Being the only day off work in the early part of the twentieth century, Sunday could be seen as a 'liberation' from the routine obligations and disciplines of work. However, as one's strongest tie to reality, work helped to regulate the unconscious mind, as a quote retrieved by Warr (1987, p71) from a 1950s book dramatically outlined:

> A considerable number of persons are able to protect themselves against the outbreak of serious neurotic phenomena only through intense work. Owing to the exaggerated repression of their impulses, they are in constant danger of having their excess excitation transformed into neurotic symptoms . . . more or less serious and acute neurotic symptoms appear if and when the work is interrupted by influences from without.

I will return to Warr's (1987) work in Chapter 7, as a basis for thinking about the task of implementing a care plan. Before leaving the subject of work, though, it is worth emphasising that the same kind of influence of a nurse's work on his or her emotional coping has been noted. Menzies (1970) suggested that in general nursing at least, the organisation of work into different tasks performed by different nurses provided emotional protection.

Economic change at the societal level is a step removed from an individual's employment status, but it also appears to have an important bearing on wellbeing. A review of admissions to a New York State psychiatric hospital, for instance, found evidence that admissions generally increased when the economy was poor and decreased when it improved. The same was true for re-admissions, and for a variety of psychologically-loaded health indicators, including alcohol abuse, heart disease, and suicide. Again, the picture of cause and effect is complex, as economic hardship may exaggerate life stressors or reduce personal coping and social support. It may also reduce society's tolerance for psychological disorder.

Political change is another factor operating at both the general social level and directly on individuals. In the UK an example has been the White Paper, *Working for Patients* (Secretaries of State, 1989), which prescribed a significant reduction in the number of hospital beds, while its successor, *Caring for People* (Secretaries of State, 1989) suggested how those with psychological difficulties should be helped in their own homes. Both of these can be seen as ways of influencing the nature of help provided to people.

Exercise 2.3: An exercise on environmental factors

The aim of this exercise is to investigate some environmental factors for yourself, in relation to a psychiatric ward.

Using the main factors in this section, prepare a checklist of important things which you might expect to find on the ward. Items to consider in relation to the 'physical' dimension could include the decor, furnishings and personal space. The checklist might also include room for your comments (or those of the nurses or clients on the ward) regarding these items.

Environmental factor	*Key items*	*Comments (including consequences of the observed factors for client care or wellbeing)*
Physical (settings)		
Social		
Other factors (for example, social class activities, resources, policies)		

Step One is to design a suitable assessment checklist by defining key items, such as noise and density. Step Two is to assess a psychiatric ward, using the checklist. This takes the form of comments on your observations: are there, for example, any changes that you might wish to suggest? (The *Ward Atmosphere Scale* (*Table 2.1* and *Figure 2.1*) represents a worked example of this exercise.)

Working with environmental factors

One understandable reaction to all these seemingly powerful and uncontrollable environmental factors is a strong sense of helplessness. After all, it is not easy to see how we might shift the economy or a government policy! But at the level of a particular service (such as CPN) or setting (for example, the ward) there are practical ways of working with these environmental factors. Indeed, since the social dimension is such a crucial factor, and since the nurse is usually the professional person who interacts most with clients in settings such as wards, there is quite a lot that can be done.

One example is the *Ward Atmosphere Scale*, developed by Moos (1976) along with the other similar scales for community settings, such as sheltered care. The *Ward Atmosphere Scale* provides a way of assessing ten key aspects of the treatment environment, as set out in *Table 2.1*.

Table 2.1 *The 10 subscales of the* Ward Atmosphere Scale (WAS) *and their definitions*

Scale	Definition
Involvement	Measures how active and energetic patients are in the day-to-day social functioning of the ward, both as members of the ward as a unit and as individuals interacting with other patients. Patient attitudes such as pride in the ward, feelings of group spirit and general enthusiam are also assessed.
Support	Measures how helpful and supportive patients are towards other patients, how well the staff understand patient needs and are willing to help and encourage patients, and how encouraging and considerate doctors are towards patients.
Spontaneity	Measures the extent to which the environment encourages patients to act openly and freely express their feelings towards other patients and staff.
Autonomy	Assesses how self-sufficient and independent patients are encouraged to be in their personal affairs and in their relationships with staff; how much responsibility and self-direction patients are encouraged to exercise; and to what extent the staff are influenced by patient suggestions, criticism and other initiatives.
Practical orientation	Assesses the extent to which the patient's environment orients him or her towards preparing for release from the hospital and for the future. Such things as training for new kinds of jobs, looking to the future and setting and working toward practical goals are considered.

Scale	Definition
Personal problem orientation	Measures the extent to which patients are encouraged to be concerned with their feelings and problems, and to seek to understand them through openly talking to other patients and staff about themselves and their past.
Anger and aggression	Measures the extent to which a patient is allowed and encouraged to argue with patients and staff; to become openly angry and to display other expressions of anger.
Order and organization	Measures how important order is on the ward, in terms of patients (how they look, what they do to encourage order) and the ward itself (how well it is kept); also measures organization, again in terms of patients (do they follow a regular schedule; do they have carefully planned activities) and staff (do they keep appointments; do they help patients follow schedules?)
Programme clarity	Measures the extent to which the patient knows what to expect in the day-to-day routine of his ward and how explicit the ward rules and procedures are.
Staff control	Measures the extent to which it is necessary for the staff to restrict patients, i.e. in the strictness of rules, and schedules, in the relationships between patient and staff, and in measures taken to keep patients under effective control.

For comparison, Moos' *Community-Oriented Programs Environment Scale (COPES)* has twelve headings with slightly different questions; his *Physical and Architectural Features* checklist considers such factors as 'social-recreational aids', for example a lounge for casual conversation, and 'prosthetic aids', such as whether a building has stairs.

These scales have great potential, as they can be used to assess an environment, pinpoint its problems, facilitate staff discussion of how these might be tackled, and finally to evaluate whether any such action removes the problems. To illustrate these uses, in one particular study (Milne, 1986), nurses and clients in a psychiatric day hospital were asked to complete the *Ward Atmosphere Scale*. Two versions were used. One asked about the 'real' ward atmosphere: how it actually is at the time of completing the form. The second asked how nurses and clients would 'ideally' like it to be in the future. Their answers allowed the production of a graph of the real and ideal ward atmosphere (see *Figure 2.1*). As in this example, there are typically several major discrepancies between the 'real' and 'ideal', which serve to highlight problems. If you study *Figure 2.1* you will see that this day hospital had difficulties

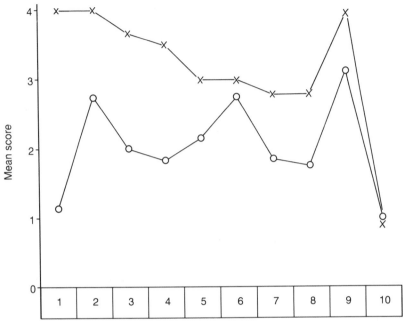

Figure 2.1 *A* Ward Atmosphere Scale *profile of a psychiatric ward. The line with crosses indicates the 'ideal' atmosphere, while the line with circles represents the 'real' or actual ward atmosphere.*

in the areas of involvement, support, spontaneity, autonomy and staff control. As a result of this assessment, staff considered these results and discussed ways of tackling them, including some staff training and a revised therapeutic programme.

The outcome of this project was a significant improvement in the ward atmosphere when it was re-assessed a few months later. This was accompanied by improvements in the clients' therapeutic gains. In other similar studies, improvements were also shown amongst the nurses, with higher morale and lower levels of absenteeism and sickness being recorded. Time and again studies based on this sort of approach have yielded similar results. This indicates that the general environment is important and that nurses *can* shape it for the benefit of themselves and their clients.

Summary

It is common sense to regard behaviour as the consequence of free will. In general, we blame people when things go wrong in their lives and praise them when things go well. However, psychology suggests that this is only half the story: a lot of behaviour would be better understood in relation to its environment. It follows that we should look at what is going on around *a client and the way in which that client interacts with his or her environment if we want to develop a sound basis for mental health nursing. To be fair, common sense also acknowledges this interplay (consider such proverbs as: 'a problem shared is a problem halved'; 'as you make your bed, so you must lie on it'; 'a burnt child dreads the fire'; 'a rolling stone gathers no moss' and so on).*

In this chapter we have considered four related dimensions of the environment and how each may impinge on our work and on our clients' wellbeing. We started from the smallest unit, the individual professional, and looked at how roles overlap and how useful distinctions might evolve. These can promote complementary specialisation within a professional group or within a team. Our next level of analysis, the multidisciplinary team, was depicted as an environment packed with difficulties and opportunities. Efforts directed at clarifying team objectives, reducing role-blurring and establishing clear lines of responsibility were seen as very worthwhile.

The next largest unit discussed was the community, which was considered in terms of the meshing of formal and informal helpers. Social support is the widespread phenomenon of such helping activities as tangible assistance and direct guidance, epitomised by the hairdressers. Voluntary organisations bridge social support and the formal help provided by the mental health professionals. We can facilitate these dimensions of help in the community, as some examples showed, and we can take account of the nature of help in relation to much of our routine work.

Lastly, I took a rather sweeping look at a very large unit, the general environment. This included such factors as the physical, social, economic and political determinants of psychological difficulty. Social class, for instance, appears to be bound up with the frequency with which certain difficulties are presented and the way in which they are treated. In turn, the living conditions of our clients play a part, as will their employment status and their social support network.

These environmental factors were not discussed in depth nor were they an exhaustive list of the important features of the context of any behaviour. But hopefully this introduction will make you more aware of the interaction between mental health and environment. As we have seen, such an awareness can significantly promote the care we provide to clients.

Questions for further consideration

1 How can distinctions be drawn between related professional groups?
2 What are the likely consequences of a lack of distinction between such groups?
3 Which guidelines are important for effective multidisciplinary teamwork?
4 Who provides what kind of psychological help, and where? For example, can you construct a 'helping profile' for your community?
5 Compare and contrast the help provided by mental health professionals with that provided by other people in the community.
6 What are the more important environmental factors influencing client behaviour?
7 How can nurses control these environmental factors for the client's benefit?
8 Where would you draw the boundaries on the client's environment?
9 Why should client behaviour change across settings?
10 How can we distinguish *cause* from *effect* in studies of the relationship between environment and behaviour?

References

Barker, P. J. (1982). *Behaviour Therapy Nursing.* London: Croom Helm.

Barrera, M., Sandler, I. N., and Ramsay, T. B. (1981). Preliminary development of a scale of social support. *American Journal of Community Psychology, 9,* 435–437.

British Association of Social Workers (BASW; 1977). *The Social Work Task.* Birmingham: British Association of Social Workers.

British Psychological Society (BPS; 1986). Responsibility issues in clinical psychology and multidisciplinary teamwork. Leicester: The British Psychological Society.

Cowen, E. (1982). Help is where you find it: four informal helping groups. *American Psychologist, 37,* 385–395.

English National Board for Nursing, Midwifery and Health Visiting (1989). *Project 2000 – A New Preparation for Practice.* Victory House, 170 Tottenham Court Road, London W1P 0HA.

Hattie, J. A., Sharpley, C. F. and Rogers, H. J. (1984). Comparative effectiveness of professional and paraprofessional helpers. *Psychological Bulletin, 93,* 534–541.

Jones, M. (1968). *Beyond the Therapeutic Community.* New Haven: Yale University Press.

Langsley, D. G. and Hollender, M. H. (1982). The definition of a psychiatrist. *American Journal of Psychiatry, 139,* 81–85.

Llewelyn, S. and Fielding G. (1983). Friction on the ward. *Nursing Mirror, 156,* March 30, 22–23.

Marshall, R. J. (1989). Blood and Gore. *The Psychologist, 2,* 115–117.

Menzies, I. (1970). *Defence Systems as Control against Anxiety.* London: Tavistock.

Milne, D. L. (1986). Planning and evaluating innovations in nursing practice by measuring the ward atmosphere. *Journal of Advanced Nursing, 11,* 203–210.

Milne, D. L., Jones, R. Q., and Walters, P. (1989). Anxiety management in the community: a social support model and preliminary evaluation. *Behavioural Psychotherapy, 17,* 221–236.

Milne, D. L., Cowie, I., Gormly, A., White, C., and Hartley, J. (1992). *Social supporters and behaviour therapists: three studies of the form and function of their help. Behavioural Psychotherapy* (in press).

Monahan, J. and Vaux, A. (1980). Task force report: the macro-environment and community mental health. *Community Mental Health Journal, 16,* 14–26.

Moos, R. H. (1976). *The Human Context: Environmental Determinants of Behaviour.* London: Wiley.

Niven, N. and Robinson, J. (1993). *The Psychology of Nursing Care: a foundation text.* Leicester: BPS Books (The British Psychological Society) and London: Macmillan.

Paykel, E. S. and Griffith, J. H. (1983). *Community Psychiatric Nursing for Neurotic Patients.* London: Royal College of Nursing.

Sanson-Fisher, R., and Jenkins, H. J. (1978). Interaction Patterns between inmates and staff in a maximum security institution for delinquents. *Behaviour Therapy, 9,* 703–716.

Secretaries of State (1989). *Working for Patients* (Cmnd 555). London: HMSO.

Secretaries of State (1989). *Caring for People: Community Care in the Next Decade and Beyond* (Cmnd 849). London: HMSO.

Shapiro, D. A. and Firth, J. (1987). Prescriptive v Exploratory Psychotherapy: Outcomes of the Sheffield Psychotherapy Project. *British Journal of Psychiatry, 151,* 790–799.

Warr, P. (1987). *Work, Unemployment and Health.* Oxford: Clarendon Press.

West, M. (1989). Visions and team innovation. *Changes, 7,* 136–140.

Willems, E. P. (1972). The interface of the hospital environment and patient behaviour. *Archives of Physical Medicine and Rehabilitation, 4,* 115–122.

Wooff, K., Goldberg, D. P. and Fryers, T. (1988). The practice of community psychiatric nursing and mental health social work in Salford. *British Journal of Psychiatry, 152,* 783–792.

Further reading

Those references listed are a mixture of general texts and detailed research studies, which you might like to pursue. In addition, here are some relevant resources:

Freeman, H. L. (Ed; 1984). *Mental Health and the Environment.* Edinburgh: Churchill-Livingstone.
Freeman's text contains chapters from experts on theory and practice (for example, on delinquency and housing).

Marks, I. M. (1985). *Psychiatric Nurse Therapists in Primary Care.* London: Royal College of Nursing.
Isaac Marks has championed the role of the nurse as specialist therapist. In this book he summarises the background to this advanced clinical role for the psychiatric nurse and then details a research study in which the work of these nurses was evaluated. This is a stimulating and positive account of psychiatric nursing in the community.

O'Connor, W. A. and Lubin, B. (Eds; 1985). *Ecological Models in Clinical and Community Mental Health*. New York: Wiley.
This text is a collection of articles which considers the relationships between context and behaviour.

Walton, H. (Ed; 1986). *Education and Training in Psychiatry*. London: King Edward's Hospital Fund for London.
This edited book contains discussion of roles and teamwork from the psychiatrist's perspective. The relationship between psychiatry and psychiatric nursing receives special attention. The tone is a constructive one in which the strengths of respective professions are emphasised.

West, J. and Spinks, P. (1988). *Clinical Psychology in Action*. London: Wright.
This edited book presents first-hand reports of what clinical psychologists do in the NHS.

Exercise 2.1: Answers
Group 1 Social Worker (British Association of Social Work, 1977)
Group 2 Clinical Psychologist (Management Advisory Service, 1989)
Group 3 Community Psychiatric Nurse (Paykel and Griffith, 1983)
Group 4 Psychiatrist (Langsley and Hollender, 1982)

Exercise 2.2: Questionnaire (see p25)
This exercise is designed to focus your understanding of social support. Complete the questionnaire that follows, then score it in order to gain an organised view of your own use of social support. You will probably find obvious differences between your uses of the different forms of support.

The Inventory of Socially Supportive Behavior
Reproduced by permission of M. Barrera. (ISSB, Barrera and Ainley, 1981)

For each of the following items, please circle the appropriate number in relation to the exercise on p25.
1 *Not at all*
2 *Once or twice*
3 *About once a week*
4 *Several times a week*
5 *About every day*

	Please circle one				
	Not at all	Once or twice	About once a week	Several times a week	About every day
During the past month, how often has somebody:					
1 Given you information on how to do something?	1	2	3	4	5

	Please circle one				
	Not at all	Once or twice	About once a week	Several times a week	About every day
2 Helped you understand why you did not do something well?	1	2	3	4	5
3 Suggested some action you should take?	1	2	3	4	5
4 Given you feedback on how you were doing without saying whether it was good or bad?	1	2	3	4	5
5 Made it clear what was expected of you?	1	2	3	4	5
6 Given you information to help you understand a situation you were in?	1	2	3	4	5
7 Checked back with you to see if you followed the advice you were given?	1	2	3	4	5
8 Taught you how to do something?	1	2	3	4	5
9 Told you who you should see for assistance?	1	2	3	4	5
10 Told you what to expect in a situation that was about to happen?	1	2	3	4	5
11 Said things that made your situation clearer and easier to understand?	1	2	3	4	5
12 Assisted you in setting a goal for yourself?	1	2	3	4	5
13 Told you what he or she did in a situation that was similar to yours?	1	2	3	4	5
14 Told you how he or she felt in a situation that was similar to yours?	1	2	3	4	5

Exercise 2.2 *Continued*

	Please circle one				
	Not at all	Once or twice	About once a week	Several times a week	About every day
15 Told you that he or she feels very close to you?	1	2	3	4	5
16 Let you know that he or she will always be around if you need assistance?	1	2	3	4	5
17 Told you that you are OK just the way you are?	1	2	3	4	5
18 Expressed interest and concern in your well-being?	1	2	3	4	5
19 Comforted you by showing you some physical affection?	1	2	3	4	5
20 Told you that he or she would keep the things that you talk about private?	1	2	3	4	5
21 Expressed esteem or respect for a competency or personal quality of yours?	1	2	3	4	5
22 Stayed with you (physically) in a stressful situation?	1	2	3	4	5
23 Listened to you talk about your private feelings?	1	2	3	4	5
24 Agreed that what you wanted to do was right?	1	2	3	4	5
25 Let you know that you did something well?	1	2	3	4	5
26 Did some activity with you to help you get your mind off things?	1	2	3	4	5

	Please circle one				
	Not at all	Once or twice	About once a week	Several times a week	About every day
27 Talked with you about some interests of yours?	1	2	3	4	5
28 Joked with you to try to cheer you up?	1	2	3	4	5
29 Gave you over £25?	1	2	3	4	5
30 Gave you under £25?	1	2	3	4	5
31 Lent you over £25?	1	2	3	4	5
32 Lent you under £25?	1	2	3	4	5
33 Provided you with a place to stay?	1	2	3	4	5
34 Lent or gave you something (a physical object other than money) that you needed?	1	2	3	4	5
35 Provided you with some transport?	1	2	3	4	5
36 Gave you some practical help with something that needed to be done?	1	2	3	4	5
37 Went with you to someone who could take action?	1	2	3	4	5
38 Provided you with a place where you could get away for a while?	1	2	3	4	5
39 Looked after a family member when you were away?	1	2	3	4	5
40 Watched over your possessions while you were away?	1	2	3	4	5

To obtain your score for each type of support add together the first 12 items (which gives the informational support score), items 13–28 (the emotional support score) and then the remaining 12 items (practical support). This will probably yield a picture of differing amounts of each type of support. It is useful to list the people who provide you with these kinds of help, and to rate how adequate your support is in relation to your needs.

SECTION TWO

Assessment

3 *The assessment process*

All the models used by the mental health professions have one thing in common: they are based on a process of assessment. For some this is subtle and complex, while for others it is relatively straightforward and clear cut. Whichever approach is used, these processes reflect the ways in which clinicians tackle the two main tasks in assessment, namely those of establishing a therapeutic relationship and of gathering relevant information. For some models these two tasks will be inseparable, while for others there may be a period of relationship-building before any attempt is made to gather information.

However, as almost all models will start off the assessment process with some kind of introduction to the working relationship between therapist and client, we will deal with this topic first. In particular, we will be concerned with those things that nurses can do to facilitate their relationship with the client. The next section addresses the question: what is assessment? I consider such issues as objectivity and measurement, citing examples of assessment methods which seem valuable in mental health nursing. I then move on to review the assessment procedure: that is, the steps we would normally follow in conducting an assessment. These steps are set out in general problem-solving terms, and we focus here on the two assessment steps of identifying and analysing a problem.

The fourth and last section takes another look at the assessment process. It looks behind the notion of 'problems' to the factors which lead people to become clients. The complexity of this process is considered in terms of the notion of 'needs': the ways in which clients, carers, staff and others define someone as meriting professional help. This again indicates the importance of the context in understanding clients, and so provides continuity with the last chapter.

What is 'assessment'?

Dictionary definitions of assessment are typically related to taxation and profit, as in 'assessable income'. The closest dictionary term to mental health nursing's definition is 'value', that is, concerned with the worth of somebody or their behaviour. Just like a balance sheet with its costs and benefits, an assessment considers a client's 'worth' in terms of strengths and weaknesses. As always, the different therapeutic models will have a variety of perspectives on assessment, but they will share the notion that it is a necessary preliminary to therapy, enabling us to understand the distinctive blend of strengths and weaknesses of each client. Once the required level of understanding is reached, the therapist decides whether to proceed to therapy and how to structure it. The decision to proceed is a complex one, as we will see in the last section of this chapter. Essentially the therapist has to consider the client's needs and the therapist's own ability to meet them.

This process of assessment leads to a quite different picture of an individual from the one that we would obtain when attempting to reach a diagnosis in the traditional psychiatric sense. In particular, these types of assessment differ in the extent to which they portray the individual as a unique person, rather than a member of a category or diagnostic group, such as 'schizophrenic'. This is just one of the many important implications of an assessment approach.

A definition of assessment

Assessment is characterised by the *systematic* way in which the clinical information is gathered. This typically involves following a careful sequence of steps, including a review of the original assessment information in the light of therapy process. It is also *thorough*, in the sense that a wide range of information is sought. *Objectivity* is another characteristic of sound assessment. This may mean using scientifically-developed methods of assessment (such as intelligence tests) when these are appropriate, or it may simply mean that the assessor's task is to be sufficiently detached from the client's distress in order to form a balanced view of the difficulty.

Validity and reliability

Objectivity is a major issue in assessment. Two main criteria for objectivity are the removal of bias (validity) and reliability.

Validity

An assessment should not be biased in any significant way. The information obtained from a client by one nurse should be the same as that obtained by another nurse assessing the same person. Psychological assessments such as the intelligence (I.Q.) tests are a good example of how such bias can be reduced, since they provide a carefully controlled situation in which the assessor follows a strict procedure. In addition, these tests provide clear rules for the interpretation of assessment information, further reducing any bias in the assessor. Bias comes in

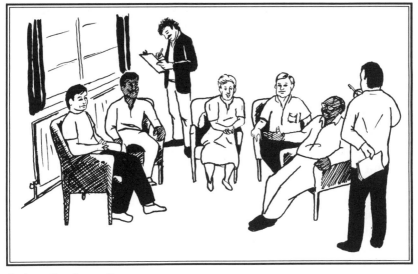

Systematic observation

many forms, such as selectively attending to certain parts of a client's behaviour while ignoring others, because one expects to observe certain things. This may be on the basis of a diagnostic label or from something someone has said about the client. A person's accent, gender or race may also introduce bias into our assessments, as we may have built up associated expectations. These sorts of biases may not be conscious, but they can considerably distort our assessment information. The general term for this criterion of objectivity is 'validity'. An assessment is said to be valid when it measures what it is supposed to measure.

In the physical world validity is a relatively straightforward matter. External factors such as a person's height, eye colour or weight can be measured by instruments, and there is no reason to question the results. In psychology, validity is a thorny problem, since many of the things we are trying to assess are internal. How can we be sure, for instance, that when we are trying to measure anxiety we really are measuring anxiety and not something else, such as fear or depression? Are the things our clients say about themselves to be taken at face value? We will return to these validity questions in Chapter 4.

Exercise 3.1: An exercise in objectivity
In order to encounter some of these objectivity problems first hand, try observing someone's behaviour at the same time as a colleague does. Before you start, agree on some things you wish to assess, such as a client's mood or a tutor's enthusiasm, and spend an agreed period doing this

completely independently. Then spend a few minutes deciding on your conclusions before comparing notes with your colleague. You will very probably disagree on some aspects of what you have observed, and possibly also on one or two of your conclusions.

Reliability

The second criterion of objectivity concerns the reliability of our assessment. If we are confident that we have a valid way of measuring a client's strengths and weaknesses, then we also want to be sure that when we conduct our assessment we get a consistent result. To return to the example of an I.Q. test, for it to be reliable we should get the same score each time we assess the same client. There should be very little fluctuation as a result of either the test or the administration of the test; any variation should be due to changes in the client. This is easily visualised if you think of a measuring tape made of elastic. Stretching it by different amounts would produce different results every time it was used to measure someone's height, and anyone else trying to use this tape would probably obtain a different height. The elastic tape would therefore be *unreliable* (each new assessment yields a new result), although it would be *valid* – it still measures height, as it is intended to do.

While it is uncommon to find reports of the reliability or validity of an interview, other assessment methods are normally accompanied by such details. Good examples are psychometric tests (for example I.Q. and personality tests), paper and pencil assessments (for example, questionnaires covering depression and anxiety) and observational schedules. I will discuss these methods again in the next chapter. For the present I will focus on illustrations of reliability and of validity.

Examples of reliability and validity in assessment instruments

The *Inventory of Depressive Symptomatology* (*IDS*; Rush *et al.*, 1986) will serve as our reliability example. The *IDS* was designed to measure specific signs and symptoms of depression in a wide range of clients. The 30-item form can be completed as a self-report questionnaire by the client, or completed by the clinician during an interview. Each question has four possible answers, and these are given scores between zero and three. For instance, the first item concerns sleep onset, and the possible answers range from 'Never takes longer than 30 minutes to fall asleep' (scores zero) to 'Takes more than 60 minutes to fall asleep, more than half the time' (which scores three). A client's score can therefore range between 0 and 84, thus giving a sensitive impression of the client's depression. The full *IDS* (Clinician-rated) is given in *Appendix I* to this chapter.

Rush *et al.* (1986) calculated the reliability of the *IDS* by comparing clients' scores throughout the administration of the instrument, the so-called *split-half method*. Scores obtained on one half of the assessment are compared with the scores from the other half (usually all odd-numbered questions compared with all even-numbered ones). A statistical test is then carried out to determine the degree of association between the two halves. If the instrument is reliable then there will be a high correlation. Rush *et al.* (1986) found a high association for the *IDS*, and on the basis of this were able to claim that the instrument was reliable.

There are several other ways of determining the reliability of an assessment. The most commonly used is to repeat the assessment at a later date and compare the two sets of results. This is called *test-retest reliability* and is often used to judge the reliability of an observational assessment.

As an illustration of how validity may be established, I will now consider a questionnaire designed to assess obsessions and compulsions. The *Padua Inventory* (Sanavio, 1988) asks clients to rate a list of 60 items for how often they are disturbed by them. Each item is rated on a five-point scale between 'not at all' (scores zero) and 'very much' (scores four). The *Padua Inventory* is reproduced in *Appendix II* to this chapter.

Sanavio (1988) looked at the validity of the *Padua Inventory* by comparing it with similar questionnaires which had been validated previously. Again, a correlation was calculated and the association was found to be high with other measures of obsessions and compulsions. On the other hand, the *Inventory* had a low correlation with a questionnaire measuring fear. Both of these findings provide some validation for the *Padua Inventory*, showing that it does seem to measure the same thing as other instruments designed to gauge obsessions and compulsions. It also discriminates between these complaints and general anxiety. These two forms of validity are called *concurrent* and *discriminant* validity.

There are several other ways of considering the validity of an assessment. The two main alternatives to the ones already considered are *content* and *construct* validity. Content validity focuses on the appropriateness of the questions included in the assessment effort, and this can be judged by the clients or by experts. For example, an interview which is supposed to assess obsessions and compulsions but which includes no questions on the client's fear of 'contamination' would be judged invalid. Construct validity, by comparison, is concerned with the extent to which an assessment instrument actually manages to measure something that is subjective. In psychology there are many things that cannot be observed directly, but which are regarded as important. Panics, dreads, worries, beliefs, neuroticism, and intelligence are cases in point. They are called *theoretical constructs*, in that they are used as a way of making sense of the things we can observe. But since we cannot see them, we may have some grounds for doubting that they actually exist. Construct validity is a way of trying to reduce our doubts, based on gradually accumulating information from other sources. For instance, the changes which take place during the rehabilitation of a long stay client should yield progressive changes in an assessment measuring their independence. If the assessment test produced a constant score over a period of rehabilitation, we would question its construct validity. We can also consider how the scores we obtain for our construct either agree or disagree with other known indicators. In this sense the *Padua Inventory* was validated by its agreement with other measures of obsessions and compulsions, and by its disagreement with measures of other kinds of constructs, such as fear and extraversion.

The feasibility and utility of assessment tools

There are two further criteria which should be mentioned briefly before I conclude this section on assessment. The first is the feasibility of the practical part of an assessment exercise. One can imagine, for instance, a situation where a structured interview or test is very time-consuming to undertake, or where special training is required to administer a rating scale, or where it is not clear how to score or interpret the results from an assessment device. These sorts of practicalities can severely hamper our use of highly valid and reliable methods.

The other criterion concerns the practical usefulness (utility) of an assessment exercise. To illustrate, a questionnaire could be reliable, valid and practical to use, yet the results it yields may have little or no bearing on the subsequent therapy. 'Good' assessment methods also have to meet this 'utility' criterion. The acid test of utility is whether the information gathered by an assessment tool or procedure helps to guide therapy towards better results. To illustrate, James *et al.* (1990) were able to demonstrate that information from assessments using the *Ward Atmosphere Scale* was useful in guiding nurses in making changes to the running of their ward. Group discussion of these results proved to be better than simply providing copies of the findings.

The assessment procedure

At the start of this chapter I considered a 'stage' view of the therapy process, in terms of a general problem-solving approach. From this perception, all therapy models essentially begin with Stage One (identification of a problem) and end with Stage Five (evaluation). While this is a helpful outline, we need more detail if we are to proceed efficiently through an assessment of a client. Indeed, there is important work to be done even before the 'problem' is identified. Whether one is about to assess an individual, a couple, a family, or a group, there is a need for preparation, to negotiate the therapeutic relationship and to agree on the tasks you all face. The comments which follow refer to able, compliant clients. It is recognised that some clients, for example those with a dementia, will not be amenable to all these points, and so some alterations will have to be made, such as agreeing needs and goals with a carer. However, the following section sets some ideal standards which should serve as reference points.

Some preliminaries

Assessment work is often preceded by a request from somebody else that you see the client. In a hospital this may arise in a team meeting, while in the community a general practitioner may ask for an assessment. Even when there is no specific request, as when individualised care plans on a ward are being drawn up, the same need for preparation exists. It is useful to know, for instance, why the problem is now acute or is being tackled at this stage. Life events such as divorce or role change may also be significant, and can sometimes be ascertained from written records, referral letters or from the team members. Having this kind of information enables you not only to meet the client with some general impression of the problem, but also to go knowing something about why the assessment is needed and hence what you are looking for. Not least, you are starting to consider the client as a unique individual and your homework indicates interest and professionalism which will be communicated to the client, with definite benefits for your therapeutic alliance. Contrast this with the client who complains that he or she has already told somebody 'all about it' and clearly resents your lack of preparation, or the lack of communication in the system.

Once you have as good a grasp of the background as possible, the next step is to meet the client or clients. Starting with the introduction, it is probably a good idea initially to err on the side of formality and politeness. For many clients your meeting will be difficult, and this approach will minimise some uncertainties, such as who is supposed to do what and how you should talk to each other. Once you have given your name and title it is appropriate in some settings to explain what you are there to do, or what the ward or service that you belong to is for. At the end of this phase, check whether the client has any questions and whether they have understood what you have said. It is usually a good idea to also ask how the client feels about your meeting.

Such preliminaries can save a lot of wasted time later on, as in the case of a client who so resents being seen that they are unforthcoming in interview, or who confuses nursing with another profession and so gives a lot of unhelpful information. These difficulties are particularly pronounced when the client is physically ill, or has hearing or sight impairments.

Once you have cleared this bit of ground (and sometimes this may take more than one meeting with the client), the way in which you are going to work together can be negotiated. As mentioned in the preceding section, the two main points to cover are the process and the techniques. This may simply mean agreeing that short rather than long meetings are preferable, and deciding on the frequency of your meetings. Such things as where you will meet (are home visits relevant and feasible?) and who will be present (other members of the team?) should also be covered. It can also be helpful to sketch out the plan, perhaps saying that you want to spend a total of so many hours carrying out the assessment, or that certain tests or methods will be used to conduct the assessment (for example, observational records or questionnaires). Again, it is necessary to keep checking that the client both understands this information and is satisfied with it. As a rule, only once these preliminaries are behind you can you move onto the first problem-solving stage of problem identification. Of course there are exceptions, as in the case of those clients who cannot or will not be interviewed (for example, an elderly client with a severe dementia). But even in these cases some of the preliminaries may still be applied in one way or another: you can let a client's spouse know who you are and what you are doing to help, for example. Carpenter and Treacher (1989) provide a clear and helpful guide to these steps in relation to marital and family therapy, while Paxton *et al.* (1988) report a study in which student nurses were trained to carry out some of these steps in interviewing.

Problem identification

The definition of a 'problem' will reflect the perspective which has been adopted. There are very few actions which everyone will see as 'problems', and several things which will lead to complete disagreement. For example, is giving up your job, leaving your family and going to live in a commune a problem or a solution? For whom, and in what ways? Because such biases are so crucial to the way in which a problem is recognised and defined, the therapist has to tread very carefully. For one thing, we should be conscious of the way that our therapeutic model encourages us to define a problem. While the behaviour therapist will notice abnormalities in a client's activities, such as avoidance of feared objects, the cognitive therapist will more readily spot distortions in the way the client thinks about that avoidance. Of course it is only right that therapists define problems in terms of their own models, but we can quickly see that the 'problem' is not an objective fact.

It follows that the important thing to do in problem identification is to define a problem clearly and carefully within the context of your therapeutic model. To go back to the example of a behavioural model, the accepted definition of a problem would consist of its frequency, intensity or duration, and this would be based on observable information. So the anxious client who avoids might have his or her problem defined in terms of how often he or she approaches the feared object, how markedly he or she shows signs of anxiety such as trembling, and how much time he or she is able to spend near the feared object before having to escape. These are objective ways of defining a problem, as another nurse could readily agree with your observations. Most therapeutic models share a concern for gathering this kind of objective information.

Another important facet of this stage is simply to communicate the definition in clear language. There is a great temptation to use 'fuzzy' terms which seem to be clear and packed with information, but which on closer inspection can be seen to be very ambiguous. 'Aggression' and 'anxiety' fall into this category. A substantial amount of time should therefore be devoted to problem identification at the outset, since this is not a simple matter and it will become the reference point for all later steps in the assessment process. We will return to the matter of what information to seek in the next chapter.

Problem analysis

This second step uses the information gathered from assessment to make sense of the problem. It is at this point that the therapist uses a model to interpret, synthesise or explain what has been more objectively defined. The usual term for this step in therapy is *problem analysis* or *formulation*. So, when someone asks about your problem analysis, you are being asked to go beyond the information and to explain the problem. For example, to answer the question 'why does this problem exist?' you may say 'the client is anxious because he experienced a traumatic incident which led to phobic avoidance and in turn to an increase in his anxiety'.

Of course, formulations are not usually so simple. Indeed, one of the most common experiences in conducting an assessment is the need to go back over parts of the problem identification, as it often proves difficult to explain why the client should have a particular difficulty at a certain moment in time. Also, one's analysis will often need to change with therapy, as this phase can provide very helpful information on the nature of the problem. To take an example, drug therapies are sometimes used to diagnose: if a client does not respond to anxiolytic medication then it is argued that they are not anxious. Nurses will be familiar with these issues from the basis of the nursing process, an explicit recognition of the need to repeatedly go through the problem-solving steps in order to fully develop each step.

Another way in which the therapist can improve the problem analysis is by confirming it with the client or with significant others. See whether your emerging explanation fits with their understanding. As the formulation develops, it should also be possible to start to make predictions. These are projections into the future about how likely something is to happen. An anxious client who has told you that they have avoided getting on a bus for the past year will be unlikely to do so in the near future. When and if they attempt to do so, they will be extremely anxious and will require maximum support and preparation. Such predictions are another way of developing the formulation, as they can provide a clear-cut test of your understanding of the problem. Perhaps the best illustration of this is the scientific method. Scientists also analyse a problem and then proceed to test certain hypotheses. If these are upheld, then they are more confident that their understanding of the phenomenon under study is accurate. When the predictions are not proven, they know that they have misunderstood and so may go back a step to the problem identification stage. In this sense, for nursing to become a more scientifically-based profession it needs to emphasise problem formulation.

Just as the analysis builds on the definition of a problem, so the rest of the steps in the nursing process (or in problem-solving more generally) follow from the analysis. At this stage, nurses can start to think about how they might tackle the problem and what they might hope to achieve. It is conventional next to consider the second part, the therapy 'goals', although in clinical practice goals and methods may influence one other: there is no point in setting up goals when you know of no methods likely to achieve them, or when you have insufficient resources.

Goal setting

Goals are an extremely useful device in therapy. They can give direction and increase motivation, and they allow evaluation to take place. However, like any powerful method, they can also work against the client's motivation. For instance, goals which are imposed by the therapist without due consultation with the client invite resistance, as do goals which are applied to everyone. Whenever possible, goals need to be discussed and agreed with the client to ensure that they are acceptable.

Goals should also reflect what is possible. They should be set with reference to what the client can realistically be expected to achieve in a given period, as well as to what the therapist (or unit or service) can reasonably be expected to provide. 'Negotiation' is the byword. This explicitly involves the client in taking responsibility and control, while simultaneously reflecting an adult relationship between therapist and client. To return to the therapeutic alliance, it is not hard to see how goal-setting in this manner cements the relationship between therapist and client.

The process of evaluation is based on goals, and can be defined as judging the extent to which goals are achieved. To follow through the nursing process to the evaluation stage therefore necessitates some clear goals. This emphasises again how each stage in problem-solving is dependent on all the other steps.

Needs assessment

As mentioned earlier, it is not easy to identify mental health problems. They are not like physical problems, as they are often demonstrated only by subjective accounts with no overt signs of difficulty. Indeed, many clients say that they wish that they did have something like a broken arm in plaster as clear evidence of their distress. One of the difficulties with mental health problems, then, is their typically private nature. Even the more conspicuous ones, such as compulsive checking rituals, may not seem particularly problematic to the observer, although acutely distressing to the sufferer.

Another difficulty with mental health problems is deciding when they exist. To illustrate, many people are known to have the kind of irrational and intrusive thoughts that characterise an 'obsessional-compulsive disorder' (OCD) or to have things in their lives that they avoid with all the intensity of a phobia. But generally they do not see this as a 'problem' and they do not seek help. When they do, the therapist may not feel that therapy is warranted, perhaps because there are judged to be more needy clients. Equally, there are clients who have little or no insight into their 'problem', but therapists (or the general public) have no difficulty in agreeing that help is needed. To this may be added the way in which members of different cultures define and present problems, not to mention gender differences within cultures. As this outline suggests, there are several parties with their own views on 'problems'.

'Problems' as 'needs'

The way that we speak about things colours the way we think about them. In turn, this is reflected in the way we tackle things, such as our job and how we feel about it. Thus, to use terms like 'problem' says quite a lot about the way a nurse is thinking. It indicates, for instance, a view in which the client is responsible for their difficulty ('it's your problem') and that it is due to a deficiency or weakness in the individual ('why can't you pull your socks up like everyone else?'). It is essentially a negative or punitive way of thinking.

The alternative perspective is to see distress or deviance in terms of needs. We all have needs after all, so it is not abnormal or weak to express them or to have other people help you to meet them (think of the needs children have, which are met by their parents). Basically, a need is 'normal' and a problem is 'abnormal'. A need is a positive way of thinking about our tasks with clients. Whereas 'problems' are often end-of-the-road conclusions with a negative damning overtone, needs are challenges or opportunities for positive, constructive change. They specify what is to be done, and so, like goals, they give direction and impetus.

Definition of a 'need'

The term 'need' can refer to a state of want or destitution, a condition requiring aid, or an imperative call or demand for some provision. As Brewin *et al.* (1987) point out, these definitions do not make it clear whether any action is actually necessary, or whether it is likely to be effective. For example, a client may have difficulty in coping but there may be nothing than can be done to help. Some researchers use the term 'need' in the same sense as 'problem', while others use it to set out the required services or help. But as the example indicates, not all problems translate into needs. From a health service perspective it will often be more useful to define needs in terms of the help required. Therefore, with Brewin *et al.* (1987), I will regard a need as the point when a client's functioning falls below some specified minimum level, and can be corrected by some course of action by the nurse or mental health service.

How are the needs identified? Here we return to the questions inherent in mental health difficulties: who decides when something merits help? It is useful to distinguish amongst the different ways in which a need is defined. It can be defined by the client or by the nurse. For the client, a distinction can also be made between 'felt need' and 'expressed need'. The former is known only to the client, whereas an 'expressed need' is a public communication. There are also two dimensions to nurses' needs assessment. One is termed *normative* and refers to the judgements made by mental health professionals such as psychiatrists and social workers, who may decide that someone is 'mentally ill' and should receive help, whether or not the client thinks so. The second dimension is called *comparative need*, in which therapists compare a client with other individuals in order to decide on the degree of need.

Unlike the other three ways of thinking about 'needs', the comparative approach is more objective, in the sense that it uses standardised tests or rating scales. The *Clifton Assessment Procedures for the Elderly* (*CAPE*; Pattie and Gilleard, 1979) for example, includes a behaviour rating scale which measures behaviour disability and results can be used to indicate dependency grades and likely need for care.

The *CAPE* score is based on clear and carefully selected areas of client functioning, such as confusion and continence, which is why it can yield an objective picture of the client. However, it is important to realise that this picture should not directly or automatically lead to conclusions about the provision of help. Between this kind of statement about client functioning and the decision about help lies a judgement. Various other factors will influence this judgement, including a clinician or carer's views about help; the extent to which the client regards their level of functioning as disabling; the kind of help that is actually available to the client in their locale; and the extent to which an environment helps or hinders a client's coping.

An example of needs assessment

Brewin *et al.* (1988) reported the results of a survey of needs amongst 145 long-term users of psychiatric day hospitals and day centres in Camberwell, London. The survey was an assessment of comparative need, based on information derived by structured interview with the client and interviews with staff, amongst other sources. They attempted to use this information to class the clients' needs, as summarised in *Table 3.1*. Their benchmark was a 'minimal level of functioning', which was derived from a list of symptoms, behaviour problems, and personal and social skills (for example, violence to others and personal cleanliness). Lists of this kind will be considered in detail in the next chapter.

On the basis of applying these categories, Brewin *et al.* (1988) were able to estimate the proportion of clients with different kinds of needs. These are listed in *Table 3.1*, with approximate percentage figures. The survey results indicated that most of these clients' needs were being met, but it also served to highlight how services might best develop in the future. For instance, they found that amongst the types of intervention provided, there was an over-provision of drugs (often they were prescribed long-term and were not reviewed) but an under-provision of psychological and educational help such as skills training. In short, careful needs assessment of this kind can indicate the task that nurses and other professionals face and highlight some of the more promising avenues for intervention.

Table 3.1 *A breakdown of comparative needs (Brewin et al., 1988). Clinical needs include 'psychotic' and 'neurotic' symptoms, while social needs include shopping and occupational skills*

Category	Proportion of sample with clinical and social needs	Definition (examples)
1. 'No need'	68%	Client's level of functioning above the minimum; no threat of relapse.
2. 'Met need'	25%	Client's level of functioning recently below the minimum.
3. 'Unmet need'	2%	Client's functioning is below the minimum and no help or only partial help has been provided.
4. 'Future need'	1%	Client is functioning below the minimum level but cannot receive any immediate help (for example, because of other priorities).
5. 'Overprovision'	3%	Help has been provided at a similar level or intensity over a long period (that is, at least two years) without altering the client's need.
6. 'Possible need'	1%	Client's may have been competent and were not currently receiving any help. However, they may subsequently need help to restore functioning.

As this example shows, 'problems' can be defined in different ways. Brewin *et al.* (1988) did not attempt to present alternative views of the 'problem', but had they done so they would probably have found considerable disagreement. To illustrate, Woods and Britton (1985) summarised some research studies conducted with elderly people in which the *functional level* or problem, did not predict the need for help. They reported that lack of self-care skills, physical disability and aggression did not necessarily signify a need for help, nor did the general degree of the dementia. It was difficult for staff to judge which problems caused the most difficulty to the carers of these elderly people, although staff were able to predict which carers were under most strain. Wood and Britton speculated that staff or carers' expectations of the client and the meaning that they give to 'problems' are probably amongst the factors influencing judgements of 'need'.

The nurse–client relationship

How do we carry out an assessment? How should the nurse and client relate to one another? How might this be facilitated? Such questions take us to the heart of the helping process, a topic of great interest to nurses and therapists over many years.

The most popular term for the nurse–client relationship is the 'therapeutic alliance'. This has been defined in the nursing context as:

> a prolonged relationship between a nurse and a client, during which the client can feel accepted by the nurse as a person of worth, feels free to express himself without fear of rejection or censure, and enables him to learn more satisfactory and productive patterns of behaviour (cited in Kagan, 1985, p239).

This definition encapsulates two points made by others, namely that a therapeutic alliance is based on an emotional bond and on the mutual involvement between nurse and client. This entails working together in the assessment of a problem. Its roots lie deep in the psychoanalytic model of psychotherapy. According to this approach, the therapeutic relationship is a necessary condition for successful help. In this model the therapist is more than an attentive listener, attempting in addition to reconstruct the atmosphere of childhood. This requires the client to relate to the therapist as he or she has done to significant others in the past (especially to parents). For example, the client may be excessively submissive and unassertive towards the therapist, because a parent insisted he or she behaved in this way towards them. Only if this kind of emotional atmosphere is generated through the therapeutic relationship will clients be able to re-experience and reconsider the way in which they have viewed themselves and others. In addition, analysts believe that clients obtain a vital sense of security from this relationship, because the therapist accepts them regardless of their actions or emotions.

The essential features of this 'analytic atmosphere' are that the therapist listens very carefully to what the client is saying in an effort to understand what is being said, particularly the emotional undercurrents. The therapist is respectful, accepting, and does not evaluate, condemn or criticise. In short, the therapist's own emotions are minimised. This usually has the effect of allowing the client to focus on his or her own emotions. It also promotes a sense of trust in the therapist, but will provoke irrational emotions, as when clients relate to the therapist as if the therapist were their parent. Such irrationality lies at the heart of psychoanalysis, since it gives the therapist information from the client's unconscious about historic difficulties within their key relationships. Freud describes this alliance as the 'best instrument' of cure.

Strupp (1973) provides a summary of the analytic perspective of the alliance in a very readable and wide-ranging textbook.

The client-centred approach

Since the early impetus provided by the analysts, several other groups have tried to develop our understanding of the therapeutic alliance. In particular, Carl Rogers and the 'client-centred' therapists have conducted much research. This dates from Rogers' (1951) famous statement that the relationship itself was a sufficient vehicle for therapeutic success. Six therapeutic 'conditions' were identified as forming this powerful relationship. They were 'empathy', 'genuineness', 'respect', 'warmth', 'concreteness' and being 'nonjudgemental'. *Empathy* refers to the ability to understand things from the other person's perspective. It has special relevance to the way clients feel about themselves and others. *Genuineness* concerns the quality of being oneself, of being natural and unaffected. Feeling comfortable with oneself as a therapist would tend to be associated with genuineness. Another sign is openness (or nondefensiveness). *Respect*, sometimes referred to as *unconditional positive regard*, is the acceptance and valuation that the therapist accords the client. A distinction is often drawn between people and their actions. Thus, although a nurse may reject or criticise a client's actions, they would not reject the client as a person. *Warmth* refers to an accepting, supportive manner, while *concreteness* is a focus on real events and on what is possible. Finally, the *nonjudgemental* attitude of

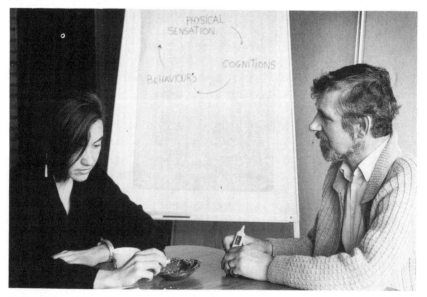

Giving information in a counselling session

the therapist is evident in the minimal use of words such as 'should' and 'ought', personal opinions and moralising.

Client-centred therapists have used a range of techniques to express these 'core conditions'. Like the analysts, the first and foremost of these is 'attending' or listening carefully to the client. Indeed it is more than words, being also the nonverbal communication of listening (for example, facial expression and eye contact). They also share an onus on being neither judgemental nor evaluative. However, a distinctive technique used by the client-centred therapists is 'reflecting'. This involves checking back with the client that you have understood the idea or feeling that is being communicated. The therapist may restate or summarise in order to aid the client's understanding of what they have been saying. These techniques may go beyond what has actually been said, when the therapist feels that this is useful. For example, a therapist may say that he or she gets the feeling that the client is very angry, although the client may not have used any emotionally-loaded terms. Further details and examples can be found in Kingston (1987). *Table 3.2* provides a summary of those counselling skills which would be expected to facilitate the therapeutic relationship, in the form of a record sheet.

Table 3.2 *A scale for recording counselling skills (to be used in the learning exercise for the therapist–client relationship)*

Counsellor skills	*Record of counsellor's speech (count or make notes)*
1. **Goal setting:** any counsellor suggestions for action that the client or the client and counsellor can take; exploration of alternatives; plans for the client; ability-potential statements that imply what the client can do to help alter the situation, change the behaviour, or get different outcomes. Most such statements include a behaviour or action for the client to try.	
2. **Confrontation:** any statement by the counsellor that calls the client's attention to something of which the client may not be aware; a statement that challenges the client, points out discrepancies in client communications, or offers a point of view different from the client's.	

Table 3.2 *Continued*

Counsellor skills	Record of counsellor's speech (count or make notes)

3. **Reflection/restatement**: counsellor statements that repeat the client's words or rephrase the content or feeling message of the client's statements.

4. **Interpretation/summary**: counsellor statements that go beyond restatement/reflection and pull together several parts of the client's content. They may or may not place any interpretation on this content.

5. **Structuring statements**: any statement that describes or explains the counselling process, places a time limit on the session, refers to physical aspects of the session such as room location, taping and so on, or is intended to give reassurance or establish rapport with the client.

6. **Probe**: any question or statement that provides a lead, seeks to clarify, or seeks to obtain information.

7. **Minimal verbal responses**: short statements indicating that the counsellor is listening and following the client's statements (for example 'um hmm', 'uh huh' or 'ok').

8. **Self-disclosure**: any statement in which the counsellor reveals own feelings, describes own experiences or shares personal data with the client.

9. **Information giving**: any statement in which the sole purpose is to pass on information to the client in the form of facts, data, resources, and so on.

10. **Other**: any miscellaneous events, not classified above (list if possible).

The role of the therapeutic alliance

Although some therapists, such as Rogers, believe that the quality of the therapeutic alliance is the main factor to consider when trying to understand why clients improve, most of them recognise that the techniques a therapist uses are also important. In general, research suggests that roughly equal contributions are made by the therapy techniques and by the therapeutic process (Chapter 6 deals with this in more detail). However, one of the unresolved puzzles is the recurring finding that despite clear differences in the theories, techniques, and, to a lesser extent, processes, associated with each model of therapy, the results they all achieve are strikingly similar (Stiles *et al.*, 1986). Chapter 9 resumes our consideration of this puzzle.

Research into the 'therapeutic conditions' has also been inconclusive. For example, while there is some evidence that these conditions are necessary for therapeutic gain, there is also evidence that such gains can be made without any contact whatsoever with a therapist. An illustration is the self help package used in anxiety management. Also, despite differences in the therapeutic processes, the results are strikingly similar. Because of these difficulties in demonstrating a clear role for therapeutic 'alliances' or 'conditions', researchers have started to consider other ways of studying the therapeutic relationship. Two interesting examples are to consider significant events in therapy sessions and to look at therapy process in terms of a series of stages. The 'significant events' approach starts from the assumption that the best predictors of therapy outcome are the client's (rather than therapists') perceptions of the therapeutic relationship. It works by asking clients to complete a brief questionnaire at the end of each therapy session. This asks them to describe the most helpful event that occurred during the session, together with any other important events (including unhelpful events). In a study introducing this approach, Llewellyn *et al.* (1988) found that clients regarded the therapist's help in increasing their awareness and in problem-solving to be the most valuable events. Reassurance and personal contact were also regarded as helpful aspects of the therapy process. Unhelpful features were the intrusion of unwanted thoughts, the imposition of unwanted responsibility and misdirection.

The stages of therapy have also been regarded as a promising way of studying the therapeutic process. While the significant events approach looks at the therapeutic process in considerable detail, the 'stages approach' takes a general overview of therapy process. This perspective stems from the observation that all therapies are a form of problem-solving, involving five stages. These stages are: problem identification, problem analysis, goal-selection, implementation of the proposed problem solution, and evaluation of the effectiveness of the therapy.

(These are very similar to the four elements of the nursing process, indicating that it too belongs to the problem-solving category). To the extent that all therapists go through these five stages, we see that they may all be similar in an important respect. So, despite the apparent differences stressed by the advocates of the various models, at the level of the therapy stages they may essentially be the same. The example just given indicated how analytic and client-centred therapists employed some similar and some dissimilar techniques for fostering the therapeutic alliance. This seems to indicate that they are related but different therapies. However, they may both proceed through the five problem-solving stages and hence be more similar than their adherents would care to concede.

More research should illuminate these aspects of the psychotherapy process, indicating other or better ways of facilitating the therapeutic alliance. At this time it does not appear that the therapist's attempts to create 'core conditions' is a useful line of enquiry. More promising are the client's perceptions of therapy and of the therapist, and the therapeutic alliance between therapist and client. That is, like so many other findings in psychology, one has to take into account the context and recognise that elements of any context interact with each other to produce an effect. One also has to consider the evidence for and against particular view points, no matter how eloquently or powerfully they are presented.

Exercise 3.2: A counselling exercise

As an exercise in the therapeutic alliance you could try working on counselling skills in trios. Take turns to be the counsellor, the client and the observer. This does not need to be carried out in a therapeutic role, but can be based on talking about yourselves on such topics as the experience of training to become a mental health nurse, or about a hobby. The 'counsellor' attempts to use counselling techniques such as 'restating' and 'summarising', while the 'client' simply talks about what they want to discuss. The observer keeps an unobtrusive record of the 'counsellor's' speech using the scale in *Table 3.2*. After a reasonable period of time (say, 15 minutes), the exercise stops and the 'client' reports his or her perception of the 'counsellor's' performance. This can be followed by discussion of the observational record. Other issues to consider are the ways in which the 'client' worked with the counsellor (the alliance) and significant events during the exercise – was anything the counsellor did particularly helpful or unhelpful? The exercise resumes with each member of the trio taking on a new role, and continues until everyone has had a turn in each role. The value of the exercise lies in clarifying the elements of counselling and learning about their helpfulness.

Two case studies of the therapeutic alliance

The relationship between nurse and patient will vary in relation to its context. Two rather different contexts are considered here to highlight this.

The first of these is taken from a ward manager's description of his work with a mixed ward of 25 chronic residential patients. Most have a diagnosis of schizophrenia, the remainder having such difficulties as depression, mania and Korsakoff psychosis. Their age range is 56 to 80 years, and they have been in-patients from two to 36 years. Treatments over this period have included electroconvulsive therapy (ECT), lobotomy, insulin and phenothiazine medication.

In contrast to such medical treatments, the ward emphasises a humanistic, holistic approach to client care. The aim is to develop a responsible, adult culture in which clients are encouraged to take responsibility for their own actions. In this culture it is crucial that the nurse has a good relationship with the client. This develops slowly, out of friendship and mutual trust, in relation to the shared daily routines of the ward. The emphasis is on caring *about* rather than caring *for* the client, and providing emotional and informational support. The ward manager regards this trusting friendship as the necessary basis for therapeutic progress, and he illustrated its importance by reference to periods when the regular staff were absent (perhaps on holiday, or ill), during which time there is usually a lot of difficulty managing the residents, and things can almost get out of control.

In addition to this professional friendship, the ward manager regards the absence of the usual restrictions as important (for example, allowing the patients to make snacks or carry out chores themselves), allied to nursing 'common sense' and special knowledge and skills. The 'working alliance' between nurse and client is therefore given top priority, with the traditional elements of hospital care (professional skills or techniques) coming bottom of the list because they are seen to play a minor role.

A rather different angle on the therapeutic relationship was obtained by speaking to a behavioural nurse therapist. This nurse had completed the Maudsley's ENB650 specialist course in behaviour therapy, enabling her to work with a wide range of adult out-patients. These included people with anxiety, depression and obsessive-compulsive disorders (OCD). They were referred to her by GPs, psychiatrists and other professionals, and were seen in health centres in the community for weekly appointments of an hour or so duration for a period of up to six months. Since completing the course in 1986 she has developed her role in terms of the kinds of problems she addresses (for example, pain and chronic fatigue), the methods she uses (she now includes cognitive therapy) and the role she plays (increasingly supervising and teaching others). Her comments therefore refer largely to her earlier work when she had her own caseload.

The behavioural nurse therapist regarded the therapeutic relationship as an essential condition for her initial work with the client, but saw it as necessarily decreasing in importance as therapy progressed. That is, early on it was important to establish a mutual commitment to therapy so that it would get underway, but latterly it became vital that the client assumed responsibility for the therapy, attributing progress to their own understanding and efforts, rather than to the therapist. In this sense she regarded the 'emotional bond' element of a therapeutic relationship as diminishing, while the 'mutual involvement' aspect increased. The atmosphere of therapy was therefore businesslike, which the therapist likened to supervising a fellow-worker. It resembled an apprenticeship model, in which the client learns skills from the 'master' therapist before becoming competent themselves.

The initial work on the emotional bond was based on adopting a professional approach to the client, including respect, genuineness and understanding. This work was done during the first two assessment appointments, and provided the basis for trust. These qualities of the relationship were thought to emerge from such approaches as reflecting back the information received, providing a rationale for the development of the problem and for therapy, and having insight into the client's experience. Examples of the quality of the relationship were how the nurse therapist could draw on her specialist experience to predict how therapeutic assignments would work, or demonstrate 'insight' into what the client was experiencing. In addition, the significant amount of time allocated to the client and the effort devoted to therapy, demonstrated in activities such as going out with the client to help them confront feared situations, cemented the emotional bond.

However, the 'mutual involvement' aspect of the relationship was where the nurse therapist placed her greatest emphasis, in keeping with the behavioural model's stress on techniques. In this respect the client was asked to undertake 'homework' tasks, such as gradually facing up to a feared object during the week until the next appointment. The client would also be asked to maintain a record of this homework, together with ratings of its difficulty. Characteristically, each therapy session would begin with a sharing of this information, together with analysis of the 'successes' and 'failures'. In the early phase of therapy, the nurse therapist would provide considerable support, guidance and encouragement to the client so that success was maximised, but over time the client was increasingly asked to assume responsibility for progress. To illustrate, one form of guidance was for the nurse to provide information of an educational kind to the client, such as some aspect of theory which would explain something that had happened, but as therapy went on she would ask the client to recall and apply this for themselves. Another example of the move towards client autonomy was the handing over of more control on the choice of weekly objectives. A crucial feature underlying these examples was the appeal to evidence in order to judge progress. That is, the clients' records and ratings of their efforts were used as the main guide to therapy (for example, evidence of 'failure' being understood in terms of having set goals that were too ambitious). This appeal to evidence tends to enhance mutual involvement in therapy.

To summarise these two case studies, both nurses regarded the therapeutic relationship as a necessary condition for effective work, despite large differences in the kinds of clients they saw, the places where they did their work, and their respective models of mental health nursing. The emphasis on the relationship with the client was greatest for the ward manager, who regarded its development as the main task for the nurse and almost sufficient on its own as a vehicle of client improvement. The behavioural nurse therapist emphasised technique-based help, necessarily starting from a straightforward working relationship.

Summary

Assessment is a systematic and objective process of information-gathering in order to define, describe and explain clients' needs. Key elements are the reliability and validity of the assessment methods, but their feasibility and the utility of the information they provide are also important. Assessment begins with some preliminary fact-finding and a clarification of procedures with the client, leading to a statement of needs and intervention goals based on problem analysis. A successful assessment process will reflect a therapeutic alliance between nurse and client. This consists of an emotional bond between them, and joint involvement in the assessment task.

Questions for further consideration

1 What is it that makes a relationship therapeutic? Try to tease out the key ingredients, perhaps with reference to a specific client.

2 Is a therapeutic alliance enough? For which clients, and in terms of which kinds of problems?

3 What part do techniques play in therapy?

4 Why is objectivity important in assessment?

5 How can we determine that an assessment method is reliable and valid?

6 What, in your opinion, is the first step in assessment?

7 'Formulation' (or problem analysis) is the bridge between assessment and therapy. Why is this so?

8 What distinguishes a 'problem' from a 'need'?

9 Give an example of a normative needs assessment, and contrast the results with those that might be obtained by a different form of assessment.

References

Brewin, C. R., Wing, J. K., Mangen, S. P., Brugha, T. S. and MacCarthy, B. (1987). Principles and practice of measuring needs in the long-term mentally ill: the MRC Needs for Care Assessment. *Psychological Medicine, 17,* 871–981.

Brewin, C. R., Wing, J. K., Mangen, S. P., Brugha, T. S., MacCarthy, B. and LeSage, A. (1988). Needs for care among the long-term mentally ill: a report from the Camberwell High Contact Survey. *Psychological Medicine, 18,* 457–468.

Carpenter, J. and Treacher, A. (1989). *Problems and Solutions in Marital and Family Therapy.* Oxford: Basil Blackwell.

James, I., Milne, D. and Firth, H. (1990). A systematic comparison of feedback and staff discussion in changing the ward atmosphere. *Journal of Advanced Nursing, 15,* 329–336.

Kagan, C. M. (Ed; 1985). *Interpersonal Skills in Nursing: Research and Application.* London: Routledge.

Kingston, B. (1987). *Psychological Approaches in Psychiatric Nursing.* London: Croom Helm.

Llewellyn, S. P., Elliott, R., Shapiro, D. A., Hardy, G. and Firth-Cozens, J. (1988). Client perceptions of significant events in prescriptive and exploratory periods of individual therapy. *British Journal of Clinical Psychology, 27,* 105–114.

Marks, I. M., Hallam, R. S., Connolly, J. and Philpotts, R. (1977). *Nursing in Behavioural Psychotherapy.* London: Royal College of Nursing.

Pattie, A. H. and Gilleard, C. J. (1979). *Manual of the Clifton Assessment Procedures for the Elderly (CAPE).* Kent: Hodder and Stoughton.

Paxton, R., Rhodes, D. and Crooks, I. (1988). Teaching Nurses Therapeutic Conversation: a pilot study. *Journal of Advanced Nursing, 13,* 401–404.

Rogers, C. R. (1951). *Client Centered Therapy.* Boston: Houghton Mifflin.

Rush, A. J., Giles, D. E., Schlesser, M. A., Fulton, C. L., Weissenberger, J. and Burns, C. (1986). The *Inventory for Depressive Symptomatology (IDS):* pre-liminary findings. *Psychiatry Research, 18,* 65–87.

Sanavio, E. (1988). Obsessions and compulsions: The *Padua Inventory. Behaviour Research and Therapy, 26,* 169–177.

Strupp, H. H. (1973). *Psychotherapy: Clinical, Research and Theoretical Issues.* New York: Jason Aronson.

Woods, R. T. and Britton, P. G. (1985). *Clinical Psychology with the Elderly*. London: Routledge.

Further reading

Anastasi, A. (1976). *Psychological Testing*. London: Collier Macmillan.
This is a masterpiece on the wide spectrum of issues associated with testing, which is one part of assessment. It includes extended accounts of reliability and validity in a way that applies to other forms of assessment.

Barker, P. J. (1985). *Patient Assessment in Psychiatric Nursing*. London: Croom Helm.
Phil Barker is well worth reading on any subject. He looks at assessment from the nurse's perspective, considering such issues as interviewing, history-taking and the assessment of different problems.

Dexter, G. and Wash, M. (1986). *Psychiatric Nursing Skills: a Patient-Centred Approach*. London: Croom Helm.
This book takes a strongly client-centred perspective, considering how the nurse and client function first and foremost as people.

Hokanson, J. E. (1983). *Introduction to the Therapeutic Process*. London: Addison-Wesley.
The particular value of this book lies in its detailed consideration of the steps in assessment and therapy. There are many verbatim examples of what therapists within different approaches say to the client.

Kagan, C. M., (Ed; 1985). *Interpersonal Skills in Nursing; Research and Applications*. London: Croom Helm.
The contributors to this volume cover much of the detail of the therapeutic process alongside related topics.

Stiles, W. B., Shapiro, D. A. and Elliott, R. (1986). Are all psychotherapies equivalent? *American Psychologist, 41,* 165–180.
A magnificent overview of the relationship between the process and outcomes of therapy.

Strupp, H. H. (1973). *Psychotherapy: Clinical, Research and Theoretical Issues*. New York: Jason Aronson.
This is a large collection of the work of this famous psychotherapist. It is very readable and covers a wide range of questions using a combination of detailed research reports and well-reasoned arguments based on clinical experience. Amongst the issues addressed in depth are the therapeutic alliance and the analysis of what goes on in therapy.

Appendix I

INVENTORY OF DEPRESSIVE SYMPTOMATOLOGY (CLINICIAN-RATED)

NAME: (Print)   SCORE:

| MARKING DIRECTIONS | OFFICE USE ONLY Staff Initials | STUDY CODE | STUDY ID NO. | VISIT CODE | TODAY'S DATE Month | Day | Year | INTAKE ID NUMBER |

MARKING DIRECTIONS

- USE A NO. 2 PENCIL ONLY
- DARKEN THE OVAL COMPLETELY
- ERASE CLEANLY ANY MARKS YOU WISH TO CHANGE
- DO NOT MAKE ANY STRAY MARKS ON THIS FORM

USE NO. 2 PENCIL ONLY

Proper Marks
●●●●

Improper Marks
⊗ ⊘ ⊙ ◔

Months: Jan, Feb, Mar, Apr, May, Jun, Jul, Aug, Sep, Oct, Nov, Dec

SITE
C_____
E_____

Please mark one response to each item that best describes the patient for the last seven days.

1. Sleep Onset Insomnia:

- ⓪ Never takes longer than 30 minutes to fall asleep.
- ① Takes at least 30 minutes to fall asleep, less than half the time.
- ② Takes at least 30 minutes to fall asleep, more than half the time.
- ③ Takes more than 60 minutes to fall asleep, more than half the time.

2. Mid-Nocturnal Insomnia:

- ⓪ Does not wake up at night.
- ① Restless, light sleep with few awakenings.
- ② Wakes up at least once a night, but goes back to sleep easily.
- ③ Awakens more than once a night and stays awake for 20 minutes or more, more than half the time.

3. Early Morning Insomnia:

- ⓪ Less than half the time, awakens no more than 30 minutes before necessary.
- ① More than half the time, awakens more than 30 minutes before need be.
- ② Awakens at least one hour before need be, more than half the time.
- ③ Awakens at least two hours before need be, more than half the time.

4. Hypersomnia:

- ⓪ Sleeps no longer than 7-8 hours/night, without naps.
- ① Sleeps no longer than 10 hours in a 24 hour period (include naps).
- ② Sleeps no longer than 12 hours in a 24 hour period (include naps).
- ③ Sleeps longer than 12 hours in a 24 hour period (include naps).

5. Mood (Sad):

- ⓪ Does not feel sad.
- ① Feels sad less than half the time.
- ② Feels sad more than half the time.
- ③ Feels intensely sad virtually all of the time.

6. Mood (Irritable):

- ⓪ Does not feel irritable.
- ① Feels irritable less than half the time.
- ② Feels irritable more than half the time.
- ③ Feels extremely irritable virtually all of the time.

7. Mood (Anxious):

- ⓪ Does not feel anxious or tense.
- ① Feels anxious/tense less than half the time.
- ② Feels anxious/tense more than half the time.
- ③ Feels extremely anxious/tense virtually all of the time.

GO ON TO NEXT PAGE →

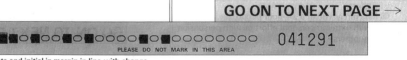

PLEASE DO NOT MARK IN THIS AREA   041291

← Changes: Date and initial in margin in line with change.

8. **Reactivity of Mood:**

⓪ Mood brightens to normal level and lasts several hours when good events occur.
① Mood brightens but does not feel like normal self when good events occur.
② Mood brightens only somewhat with few selected, extremely desired events.
③ Mood does not brighten at all, even when very good or desired events occur.

9. **Mood Variation:**

⓪ Notes no regular relationship between mood and time of day.
① Mood often relates to time of day due to environmental circumstances.
② For most of week, mood appears more related to time of day than to events.
③ Mood is clearly, predictably, better or worse at a fixed time each day.

→ **9A. Is mood typically worse in (mark one).**

    ○ morning
    ○ afternoon
    ○ night

→ **9B. Is mood variation attributed to environment by the patient? (mark one).**

    ○ Yes   ○ No

10. **Quality of Mood:**

⓪ Mood is virtually identical to feelings associated with bereavement or is undisturbed.
① Mood is largely like sadness in bereavement, although it may lack explanation, be associated with more anxiety, or be much more intense.
② Less than half the time, mood is qualitatively distinct from grief and therefore difficult to explain to others.
③ Mood is qualitatively distinct from grief nearly all of the time.

Complete either 11 or 12 (not both)

11. **Appetite (Decreased):**

⓪ No change from usual appetite.
① Eats somewhat less often and/or lesser amounts than usual.
② Eats much less than usual and only with personal effort.
③ Eats rarely within a 24-hour period, and only with extreme personal effort or with persuasion by others.

12. **Appetite (Increased):**

⓪ No change from usual appetite.
① More frequently feels a need to eat than usual.
② Regularly eats more often and/or greater amounts than usual.
③ Feels driven to overeat at and between meals.

Complete either 13 or 14 (not both)

13. **Weight (Decrease) Within The Last Two Weeks:**

⓪ Has experienced no weight change.
① Feels as if some slight weight loss occurred.
② Has lost 2 pounds or more.
③ Has lost 5 pounds or more.

14. **Weight (Increase) Within The Last Two Weeks:**

⓪ Has experienced no weight change.
① Feels as if some slight weight gain has occurred.
② Has gained 2 pounds or more.
③ Has gained 5 pounds or more.

15. **Concentration/Decision Making:**

⓪ No change in usual capacity to concentrate and decide.
① Occasionally feels indecisive or notes that attention often wanders.
② Most of the time struggles to focus attention or make decisions.
③ Cannot concentrate well enough to read or cannot make even minor decisions.

16. **Outlook (Self):**

⓪ Sees self as equally worthwhile and deserving as others.
① Is more self-blaming than usual.
② Largely believes that he/she causes problems for others.
③ Ruminates over major and minor defects in self.

17. **Outlook (Future):**

⓪ Views future with usual optimism.
① Occasionally has pessimistic outlook that can be dispelled by others or events.
② Largely pessimistic for the near future.
③ Sees no hope for self/situation anytime in the future.

GO ON TO NEXT PAGE →

18. Suicidal Ideation:

⓪ Does not think of suicide or death.
① Feels life is empty or is not worth living.
② Thinks of suicide/death several times a week for several minutes.
③ Thinks of suicide/death several times a day in depth, or has made specific plans, or attempted suicide.

19. Involvement:

⓪ No change from usual level of interest in other people and activities.
① Notices a reduction in former interests/activities.
② Finds only one or two former interests remain.
③ Has virtually no interest in formerly pursued activities.

20. Energy/Fatiguability:

⓪ No change in usual level of energy.
① Tires more easily than usual.
② Makes significant personal effort to initiate or maintain usual daily activities.
③ Unable to carry out most of usual daily activities due to lack of energy.

21. Pleasure/Enjoyment (exclude sexual activities):

⓪ Participates in and derives usual sense of enjoyment from pleasurable activities.
① Does not feel usual enjoyment from pleasurable activities.
② Rarely derives pleasure from any activities.
③ Is unable to register any sense of pleasure/enjoyment from anything.

22. Sexual Interest:

⓪ Has usual interest in or derives usual pleasure from sex.
① Has near usual interest in or derives some pleasure from sex.
② Has little desire for or rarely derives pleasure from sex.
③ Has absolutely no interest in or derives no pleasure from sex.

23. Psychomotor Slowing:

⓪ Normal speed of thinking, gesturing, and speaking.
① Patient notes slowed thinking, and voice moderation is reduced.
② Takes several seconds to respond to most questions; reports slowed thinking.
③ Is largely unresponsive to most questions without strong encouragement.

24. Psychomotor Agitation:

⓪ No increased speed or disorganization in thinking or gesturing.
① Fidgets, wrings hands and shifts positions often.
② Describes impulse to move about and displays motor restlessness.
③ Unable to stay seated. Paces about with or without permission.

25. Somatic Complaints:

⓪ States there is no feeling of limb heaviness or pains.
① Complains of headaches, abdominal, back or joint pains that are intermittent and not disabling.
② Complains that the above pains are present most of the time.
③ Functional impairment results from the above pains.

26. Sympathetic Arousal:

⓪ Reports no palpitations, tremors, blurred vision, tinnitus or increased sweating, dyspnea, hot and cold flashes, chest pain.
① The above are mild and only intermittently present.
② The above are moderate and present more than half the time.
③ The above result in functional impairment.

27. Panic/Phobic Symptoms:

⓪ Has neither panic episodes nor phobic symptoms.
① Has mild panic episodes or phobias that do not usually alter behavior or incapacitate.
② Has significant panic episodes or phobias that modify behavior but do <u>not</u> incapacitate.
③ Has incapacitating panic episodes at least once a week or severe phobias that lead to complete and regular avoidance behavior.

28. Gastrointestinal:

⓪ Has no change in usual bowel habits.
① Has intermittent constipation and/or diarrhea that is mild.
② Has diarrhea and/or constipation most of the time that does not impair functioning.
③ Has intermittent presence of constipation and/or diarrhea that requires treatment or causes functional impairment.

GO ON TO NEXT PAGE →

← Changes: Date and initial in margin in line with change.

29. Interpersonal Sensitivity:

ⓞ Has not felt easily rejected, slighted, criticized or hurt by others at all.

① Occasionally feels rejected, slighted, criticized or hurt by others.

② Often feels rejected, slighted, criticized or hurt by others, but with only slight effects on social/occupational functioning.

③ Often feels rejected, slighted, criticized or hurt by others that results in impaired social/occupational functioning.

30. Leaden Paralysis/Physical Energy:

ⓞ Does not experience the physical sensation of feeling weighted down and without physical energy.

① Occasionally experiences periods of feeling physically weighted down and without physical energy, but without a negative effect on work, school, or activity level.

② Feels physically weighted down (without physical energy) more than half the time.

③ Feels physically weighted down (without physical energy) most of the time, several hours per day, several days per week.

Changes: Date and initial in margin in line with change. ⟶

THANK YOU

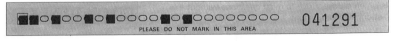

PLEASE DO NOT MARK IN THIS AREA

041291

Printed in U.S.A.   Mark Reflex® by NCS MP83431:321   A2202

Appendix II: *The Padua Inventory*

Instructions: The following statements refer to thoughts and behaviors which may occur to everyone in everyday life. For each statement, choose the reply which best seems to fit you and the degree of disturbance which such thoughts or behaviors may create. Rate your replies as follows:

0 *not at all*
1 *a little*
2 *quite a lot*
3 *a lot*
4 *very much*

1 I feel my hands are dirty when I touch money.
2 I think even slight contact with bodily secretions (perspiration, saliva, urine etc.) may contaminate my clothes or somehow harm me.
3 I find it difficult to touch an object when I know it has been touched by strangers or by certain people.
4 I find it difficult to touch garbage or dirty things.
5 I avoid using public toilets because I am afraid of disease and contamination.
6 I avoid using public telephones because I am afraid of contagion and disease.
7 I wash my hands more often and longer than necessary.
8 I sometimes have to wash or clean myself simply because I think I may be dirty or 'contaminated'.
9 If I touch something I think is 'contaminated' I immediately have to wash or clean myself.
10 If an animal touches me, I feel dirty and immediately have to wash myself or change my clothing.
11 When doubts and worries come to my mind, I cannot rest until I have talked them over with a reassuring person.
12 When I talk I tend to repeat the same things and the same sentences several times.
13 I tend to ask people to repeat the same things to me several times consecutively, even though I did understand what they said the first time.
14 I feel obliged to follow a particular order in dressing, undressing and washing myself.
15 Before going to sleep I have to do certain things in a certain order.
16 Before going to bed I have to hang up or fold my clothes in a special way.

17 I feel I have to repeat certain numbers for no reason.

18 I have to do things several times before I think they are properly done.

19 I tend to keep on checking things more often than necessary.

20 I check and recheck gas and water taps and light switches after turning them off.

21 I return home to check doors, windows, drawers etc., to make sure they are properly shut.

22 I keep on checking forms, documents, checks etc. in detail, to make sure I have filled them in correctly.

23 I keep on going back to see that matches, cigarettes etc. are properly extinguished.

24 When I handle money I count and recount it several times.

25 I check letters carefully many times before posting them.

26 I find it difficult to take decisions, even about unimportant matters.

27 Sometimes I am not sure I have done things which in fact I know I have done.

28 I have the impression that I will never be able to explain things clearly, especially when talking about important matters that involve me.

29 After doing something carefully, I still have the impression I have either done it badly or not finished it.

30 I am sometimes late because I keep on doing certain things more often than necessary.

31 I invent doubts and problems about most of the things I do.

32 When I start thinking of certain things, I become obsessed with them.

33 Unpleasant thoughts come into my mind against my will and I cannot get rid of them.

34 Obscene or dirty words come into my mind and I cannot get rid of them.

35 My brain constantly goes its own way and I find it difficult to attend to what is happening round me.

36 I imagine catastrophic consequences as a result of absent-mindedness or minor errors which I make.

37 I think or worry at length about having hurt someone without knowing it.

38 When I hear about a disaster, I think it is somehow my fault.

39 I sometimes worry at length for no reason that I have hurt myself or have some disease.

40 I sometimes start counting objects for no reason.

41 I feel I have to remember completely unimportant numbers.

42 When I read I have the impression I have missed something important and must go back and reread the passage at least two or three times.

43 I worry about remembering completely unimportant things and make an effort not to forget them.

44 When a thought or doubt comes into my mind, I have to examine it from all points of view and cannot stop until I have done so.

45 In certain situations I am afraid of losing my self-control and doing embarrassing things.

46 When I look down from a bridge or a very high window, I feel an impulse to throw myself into space.

47 When I see a train approaching I sometimes think I could throw myself under its wheels.

48 At certain moments I am tempted to tear off my clothes in public.

49 While driving I sometimes feel an impulse to drive the car into someone or something.

50 Seeing weapons excites me and make me think violent thoughts.

51 I get upset and worried at the sight of knives, daggers and other pointed objects.

52 I sometimes feel something inside me which makes me do things which are really senseless and which I do not want to do.

53 I sometimes feel the need to break or damage things for no reason.

54 I sometimes have an impulse to steal other people's belongings, even if they are of no use to me.

55 I am sometimes almost irresistibly tempted to steal something from the supermarket.

56 I sometimes have an impulse to hurt defenseless children or animals.

57 I feel I have to make special gestures or walk in a certain way.

58 In certain situations I feel an impulse to eat too much, even if I am then ill.

59 When I hear about a suicide or a crime, I am upset for a long time and find it difficult to stop thinking about it.

60 I invent useless worries about germs and diseases.

4 *Methods of assessment*

Chapter 3 focused on the way in which we go about the task of assessment, and addressed the question of *how* to assess. This chapter deals with the closely related question of *what* to assess. This includes the general strategy for gathering information about clients (through interviews or observations, for example), and it also refers to the assessment tools, such as questionnaires or record sheets that can be used to improve the information we gather. As I will point out, assessments have other dimensions, such as who assesses, and when. I will use 'method' to refer to a systematic approach to information gathering in relation to these dimensions.

Having considered these assessment dimensions I will focus on some examples of each of the main strategies and instruments. A case study will be used to show how these can be part of mental health nursing practice. In this chapter I will use a case from the work of a community psychiatric nurse, and as a result, it should be relatively easy to see how the different assessment methods can be introduced into a typical work environment.

Finally, I will weigh up the assessment methods in terms of such issues as their utility and ease of administration. For although one can readily see that certain assessment methods are 'a good thing' (providing lots of useful information in relation to minimal professional time), there are inevitably strengths and weaknesses associated with all of the methods. It is important to take these into account before deciding to use a particular strategy or technique with a client.

An outline of the assessment methods

There are a number of ways of thinking about the different approaches to assessment. The approaches can be classified by the way in which the information is gathered, such as 'self-report' or 'questionnaire'; or they can be classed in terms of the kind of client problem being assessed, such as difficulties with thoughts, feelings and behaviours. Another assessment dimension is the focus of the problem analysis, used in assessments directed at the individual, the couple, or the family. These attempt to explain why there is a problem, as in relating depression to an unsuccessful marriage. As a final illustration, assessments may also vary along the dimension of 'restrictiveness'. That is, they differ in how much the client is required to conform to assessment requirements. For example, direct observation places no constraints on the client's movements, whereas an interview requires that the client sits down in a private room and responds in a one-to-one situation over a period of time.

Although these various approaches may at first appear bewildering, the idea behind assessment methods is actually very much like that behind many other things in life. To take a close parallel, in general nursing the assessment methods also vary on restrictiveness (for example, having to keep still for an X-ray) or level of analysis (for example, biochemical assays and general self-reports of wellbeing), to take just two examples. Similarly, if we wanted to find out why a car was not working properly we might consider a number of strategies, such as electrical tuning tests, observing changes in performance in relation to changes in environment (does the car only overheat in traffic?), or by systematically testing all the relevant components. This is also how we might use a symptom checklist or questionnaire in mental health. In short, the available methods reflect the need for a range of logical strategies for defining and understanding problems.

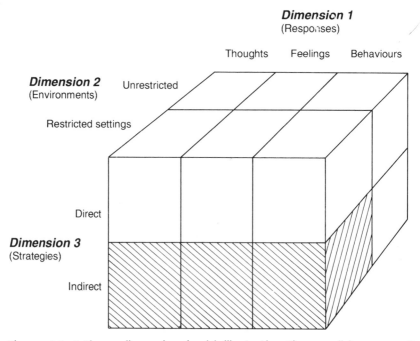

Figure 4.1 *A three-dimensional grid, illustrating the possible range of assessment approaches across responses, environments and assessment strategies.*

The 'assessment grid' (see *Figure 4.1*) is one way of summarising some of the different strategies used in mental health nursing (Cone, 1978). This shows in graphical form how we can combine several different dimensions of assessment. This particular grid shows the relationship between the three very broad dimensions of *strategies, environments* and *responses*. I have already mentioned how the assessment environment can vary in the extent to which it restricts the client. In this example strategies are broken down into *direct* and *indirect* forms. This refers to whether the client's problem is assessed in terms of behaviour (that is, by observation), or whether, in contrast, the problem is assessed by gathering information on less overt aspects of a problem. Examples of this indirect strategy would include physiological data, client self-report (including interviews) or nurses' ratings of a client's attitude to treatment.

The third dimension, labelled *responses*, considers the main ways in which a problem can be considered. These are *thoughts, feelings* and *behaviours*. Many psychiatric diagnoses are presented in these terms, although one of these may dominate for a given diagnosis. Depression, for instance, is first recognised from its feeling component, as in a client's statements of sadness, misery, despondency and hopelessness. However, there are also thinking elements (a client believing that he or she is worthless; that the future is black) and behavioural features, such as sleep disturbance, and monotonous speech.

To return to *Figure 4.1*, most assessment techniques can be fitted into one or more cells of this grid. I have hatched three cells to illustrate how we would classify an interview, structured so as to elicit information from the client about their thoughts, feelings and behaviour. As an interview is an indirect method used in a restricted setting, it belongs in the bottom corner of the assessment grid. Another technique, such as an observation schedule, would be placed in a different cell. It would be on the 'behaviours' response dimension assessed in an unrestricted setting (for example, moving around the ward) and would be a direct method. This places it in the top right hand cell.

As already mentioned, the three dimensions in *Figure 4.1* do not exhaust the assessment dimensions. This is perhaps unfortunate if you want a nice simple picture of assessment, but from a practical perspective the remaining dimensions give more assessment options. For example, one can add the temporal dimension, which addresses the question of when data are to be gathered. It is rare to gather information continuously. More commonly we 'sample' clients' difficulties, perhaps asking them how they feel at different times in the day, or in observing them closely at mealtimes. Another dimension omitted from *Figure 4.1* is the assessor. Obviously, different people can usefully contribute to an assessment picture, including the client him or herself, their family and friends, as well as the different perspectives of the members of the multidisciplinary team.

We can summarise all these dimensions by considering the following questions:

- *who* will provide information? – the assessor dimension;
- *what* will be assessed? – the triple response system dimension;
- *why* is there a problem? – dimension from inside clients to the relationship they have with others (levels of assessment);
- *where* will the assessment be conducted? – the environmental dimension;
- *when* will an assessment be conducted? – the temporal dimension;
- *how* is the information to be gathered – the strategy dimension, including *which* technique is best? – the selection of an appropriate instrument.

We can think of these dimensions as being similar to the segments of an orange (see *Figure 4.2*). Working out from the centre are the various aspects of an assessment method, with the client represented at the centre. The segments therefore represent the questions to be addressed.

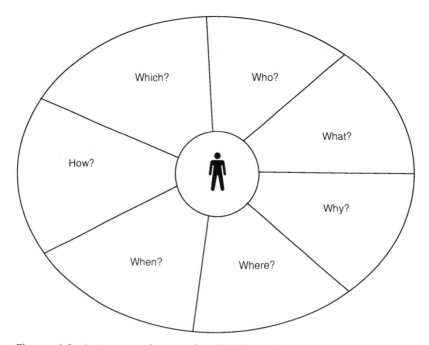

Figure 4.2 *An 'orange image' for thinking about the assessment dimensions. The client is represented by the centre, while the segments represent the dimensions.*

Having considered the general dimensions of assessment, it is now appropriate to look at some of them in more depth.

Who should provide information?

If the clients are able to contribute to the assessment then they should of course do so fully. Their perception is usually of greatest interest because they are often the originator of the referral, and because their view of the problem is itself of crucial importance. In some cases distorted perceptions are the problem. In addition, one would normally seek the views of 'significant others' (such as partners and parents) on the problem as a way of placing the client's views in some sort of context and of obtaining a range of views.

When clients are unable to provide this assistance, the views of others take on an extra significance. Florid psychoses and severe dementias are obvious illustrations, with dementias in particular being a good example of the importance of a carer's perspective. Evidence suggests that it is not the severity of the problem itself (for example, the client's wandering or incontinence) which causes the carer to call for help; rather it is the carer's own capacity to cope that is crucial. Their perception of the problem is a central feature of their coping. Research suggests that the carer's capacity for construing their task in terms of virtues (such as 'it's good to help other people, especially one's family') is one such coping strategy (Woods and Britton, 1985).

What to assess?

In general it is a good idea to consider thoughts (cognitions), feelings (affect) and behaviour (responses; action). Most problems have an impact on more than one of these dimensions. Recent psychological research has focused on the relationship between thoughts, feelings and behaviour. The technical term used to describe them is the *triple response system* or *three systems analysis* (Rachman, 1978). Studies have generally found only a small degree of overlap between these three responses, although this varies depending on circumstances. The importance of the three systems analysis is that careful assessment should consider them all, in order to discover which system shows greatest abnormality. Better treatment results may then be achieved by focusing on this system, rather than, for example, trying to address all three equally. The therapy should address the most disturbed system. Thus, if behaviour is the most abnormal element, it is addressed by behavioural techniques, such as desensitisation for avoidance of feared situations; if thoughts are most disturbed then cognitive therapies might be tried; and if feelings were identified as the most problematic system, we might introduce ways of altering the physiological state, such as progressive muscular relaxation.

The triple response approach can also help in establishing a sound base for subsequent evaluation. Just as the problem can at first present a variable picture across these three responses, so beneficial change with therapy may effect them differentially. One can imagine that a client with agoraphobia might be helped to alter negative and irrational beliefs, while still remaining housebound. They (or their partner) may then request continued help to address this behavioural aspect of their needs.

One may also usefully assess a problem in ways that extend beyond the individual, as our carer example illustrated earlier. In principle, one may be interested in how the client's problem impinges on other people at home, at work, or at play. This may further help in formulating a problem or in evaluating therapy.

Why is there a problem?

In dealing with this most difficult of questions we will often wish to appeal to clients and significant others for enlightenment. According to some therapeutic models, there is little point in raising the question, since the client's unconscious mind conceals the answer. Other models do place a value on the client's ability to explain the origin or persistence of a problem, but seek to bolster it with other information. This may be material which is known to clients, but which is not seen by them as especially significant. As a consequence, they do not volunteer it in interview. It may also be material which is fairly meaningless on its own, but which the therapist can combine with other information (and their knowledge of similar problems) to make sense of the problem. To illustrate, someone with a checking ritual (part of the 'obsessional-compulsive disorder') may readily report that they feel 'relieved' after ritualising, but not attribute any special significance to this experience. The behaviour therapist would, however, see this as a crucially important determinant of the problem, the 'escape conditioning' which maintains it.

Few problems are adequately explained in simple terms. There are usually different issues, such as the connection between life events and the problem's onset, or the association between a problem and the difficulties significant others themselves experience in coping. Some therapy models go so far as to suggest that the client may effectively represent, or carry, a family problem on the family's behalf (the *scapegoat hypothesis*). There are many books available which offer explanations for psychological problems in terms of these sorts of notion. As there is no compelling evidence on the validity of many of these explanations, it can be difficult to decide on their value.

However, one thing that many models share is the idea that a problem can best be understood at different levels. It is argued that although superficially divergent, clients' difficulties are increasingly similar at a 'deeper' level. Thus, two anxious clients may present quite distinctly, one with behavioural difficulties, the other with affective distress. But when assessed further, both may well describe a fear of fear itself (that is, of the symptoms they experience). At the next level down, they may express a dread of some impending personal disaster, and this may be the same disaster (for example, going insane). If they don't concur at this level of the problem, they may still agree on a fear of losing control, a property shared by heart attacks and going insane. Deeper down still, they may fear abandonment, a complete isolation from, and rejection by, other people.

Assessment of these underlying reasons for a problem requires special sensitivity by the therapist, but holds the key to a more adequate answer to the question 'why?' Called *laddering*, this approach can help us to understand why a range of seemingly unrelated problems go together. To illustrate, a depressed person who presents with helplessness at work may also indicate difficulties in other areas. They may have given up their hobby or started divorce proceedings. Although not necessarily tied to the work problem, these difficulties may all come together at another level of the assessment. This might be an irrational belief about their inability to influence important things, for example, 'I am unable to get anything right, so why bother with anything?' By defining 'the problem' at some such level, the therapist can better see where or how to help.

Where to assess?

Just as one would want to try to understand a problem at different levels, so one would also wish to assess it in different settings. A client's account is unlikely to ever be a 'true' reflection of a problem, because of the inevitable biases which come into play when describing oneself. In some forms of psychotherapy, such as psychoanalysis, this distortion is used by the therapist as a guide to the unconscious, seen as the determinant of the client's behaviour.

In other kinds of psychotherapy, the therapist is more interested in obtaining an objective account of the problem. To illustrate, therapists using the family therapy model might wish to observe in a structured way how family members relate to one another, and so the therapists might do their assessment (and therapy) within the clinical setting. This setting might have one-way mirrors and microphones, which allow the therapy team to follow every detail of the exchanges. At the other extreme, a therapist may wish to observe the client's activities in their own environment (for example, the client's home or work), in which case they would place little or no constraints on the client, and use few or no instruments.

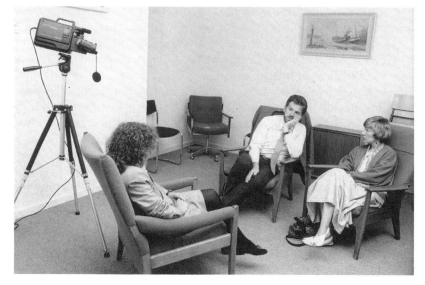

Assessment in family therapy

In essence, the therapist wishes to sample the relevant client thoughts, feelings or behaviours. This may dictate a restricted range of assessment settings, such as the psychoanalyst's traditional use of the reclining chair as the place for information to be gathered. But when the therapeutic model is concerned with more objective data, the settings that are sampled will tend to be more numerous and varied. Behaviour therapists, in contrast, might use interviews in the clinic to obtain an initial problem outline, before observing the client's behaviour in a setting in which the problem occurs. They may also make use of the role-plays in somewhat artificial settings, as illustrated by social skills training in a group convened by the therapist. In this fashion, two or more sources of information can be used to develop a picture of a problem. This will tend to improve the accuracy of the assessment and to yield more ideas about why the problem exists.

When to assess?

While it is customary to emphasise that assessment precedes therapy, in practice it makes good sense to return to an assessment phase (or to the original assessment material) during therapy. The term 'nursing process' is intended to reflect this need to go back and forth from an understanding of the problem to some form of care plan. No sooner do we think that we have a clear idea of a problem than our intervention suggests otherwise. That is, we continue to 'assess' through our therapy. This is partly because our understanding is always partial, and so can always be developed, and partly because the care plan represents a different way of looking at the client. It may, for instance, change the therapist–client relationship from a non-directive one in the assessment phase to a more directive approach during therapy.

Additionally, therapy may well entail that the client alters important parts of their world, thus generating new information. The therapist will seek to gather this and relate it to what is already known. In this sense, therapy can be seen as an 'experiment', in which the ideas from an earlier phase of assessment are tested out. Thus, if an assessment process indicated that a client lacked self-help skills, for example, shaving, the care plan might be based on the use of various physical and verbal prompts intended to promote shaving. However, in implementing this care plan it might quickly become clear that the client actually did possess the necessary skills. This would then throw us back on our assessment, suggesting that it was flawed in some way. There may have been a lack of attention to the client's motivation, for example, and what we found in carrying out the care plan was that the client could perform the task of shaving, given some encouragement. We would then alter our assessment of the problem and, very probably, our care plan. This would lead to another round of implementation (that is, testing out our latest idea), possibly leading to new information and a further refinement to the assessment and care plan. So the nursing process would continue, ideally to the point where the care plan is successful, or at least to the point where we realise that our assessment is inadequate and discontinue therapy.

The general idea is that we are pursuing a problem-solving approach, taking care to note new information which might improve our understanding or intervention. It is an *analytic* or *scientific* approach, essentially. This is rather different from a *technique-centred* approach, in which we proceed from a crude or fixed therapeutic method, such as 'all clients with 'anxiety' should receive 'anxiety management' training'.

How to assess?

The basic strategies for gathering information can be listed as follows. *Table 4.1* summarises these and provides some illustrative techniques.

- *Interviews*: these can be structured or unstructured. The former follows a pre-determined set of questions, and is intended to answer these in relation to some theory about the kind of problem that is being assessed. Unstructured interviews, in contrast, are not intended to yield specific information. They may, for instance, serve the purpose of building up a general understanding of the client, or they could be designed to increase rapport prior to a more detailed assessment.

Table 4.1 *An outline of the main assessment strategies together with some illustrative techniques*

Assessment strategy	Representative techniques	Examples	Source
1. Interview	a) Structured interview	i) Social Behaviour Assessment Schedule	Platt *et al.* (1980)
		ii) Symptom Rating Scale	Wing (1961)
2. Self-report	a) Questionnaires	i) Fear Questionnaire	Marks (1985)
		ii) Depression Inventory	Beck *et al.* (1961)
	b) Diaries and record sheets	i) ABC Record Sheet	Barker (1985)
		ii) various records and diaries	Carnwath and Miller (1986)
3. Direct observation	a) Rating scales	i) Clifton Assessment Procedure for the Elderly (CAPE)	Pattie (1981)
		ii) Problem Ratings	Marks (1985)
	b) Checklists	i) Compulsion Checklist	Marks (1986)
	c) Schedules	i) Nurses Observation Scale for In-patient Evaluation (NOSIE)	Honigfeld (1966)
		ii) Behaviour Observation Instrument (BOI)	Alevizos *et al.* (1978)

- *Self-report*: this strategy entails some form of assessment information as gathered by the client. Common examples are symptomatic questionnaires and activity diaries or record sheets. I will provide some examples shortly. Self-report may also be used to refer more generally to whatever the client says about their problem, including providing their own view about why it arose, or verbalising freely about their thoughts during a therapy session.

- *Reports by others*: often it is useful to complement self-report data with information provided by others. On other occasions it is not practically possible to obtain self-report, or the views of significant others have special value, as in the earlier example of carers of people suffering from a dementia. For such reasons we turn to reports provided by others. These can take the same form as self-report assessments, namely questionnaires, rating scales, record sheets, and interviews.

As a nurse, you may often be asked to contribute to the assessments done by other professionals in this way. For some clients you are in the best position to provide information, as when a survey of all clients is being conducted in order to gain an overall impression of a resident client group's needs. The *Clifton Assessment Procedure for the Elderly* (*CAPE*; Pattie and Gilleard, 1979) is an example. It assesses orientation, physical disability, apathy, communication and social disturbance.

- *Analogues*: it is also possible to set up assessment situations which attempt to reproduce key challenges to the client. While these are to some extent contrived, they have the advantage of promising choice information in minimal time. Examples include the social skills role-plays mentioned earlier, as well as such devices as the client's response to 'critical incidents' represented in video or written form.

- *Equipment-based strategies*: video or audio tapes may also be used to record what a client says or does. This can offer considerable advantages in terms of an objective, reproducible record, but has to be considered against the cost in time and equipment. Another example is 'biofeedback' equipment. These machines translate the client's physiological responses (for example, heart rate and muscle tension) into numbers on a dial or sounds varying in frequency. While used mostly as a part of therapy, these machines can also provide useful assessment information.

- *Observation*: clearly there is considerable observation entailed in self-report or in the reports provided by others. However, a separate strategy is justified because of the considerable range of techniques available for use by therapists. Although rating scales such as *REHAB* (Baker and Hall, 1983) entail your observations of a client, these are lumped together in a general summary score. This may combine all three response systems and information from many different situations over many months or years. In contrast, observation is used here to refer to systematic records of specific client behaviours gathered in defined settings over time. To illustrate, behaviour therapists (the main advocates of observation) make considerable use of an A–B–C record of behaviour. This requires the observer to note the *a*ntecedents and *c*onsequences of a *b*ehaviour. For example aggressive behaviour, such as shouting or throwing, may be observed alongside the things that immediately precede and follow it. These may vary, including approaches by other clients as an antecedent, and the nurse's attention as a consequence (see Barker, 1985, for additional examples). Other methods include checklists and observation schedules. Checklists identify specific behaviours and require a tick from the observer when each such behaviour is observed. For instance, a self-help skills checklist focusing on a client's behaviour at mealtimes might look like that in *Figure 4.3*.

Specific behaviours	Mon	Tue	Wed	Date Thur	Fri	Sat	Sun
1. Collects plate from servery		✓		✓	✓	✓	✓
2. Sits down at table			✓		✓	✓	✓
3. Uses knife appropriately				✓		✓	✓
4. Uses fork appropriately				✓	✓	✓	
5. Eats one mouthful at a time			✓		✓	✓	✓
6. Returns empty plate to servery					✓	✓	✓

Figure 4.3 *Example of a self-help skills checklist.*

As the imaginary client's record shows, there has been a steady improvement in the behaviours of interest, as observed and recorded by the nurse.

Observation schedules are more varied in their format than checklists. Some may share a similar breakdown into specified behaviours, but generally they require observations to be made with a high frequency, often over a shorter period and in situations with less structure than meal times. For example, the *Behaviour Observation Instrument* (Alevizos *et al.*, 1978) is designed to record a broad range of client activities in residential settings. These include 'social participation' (for example, conversing), 'unusual or maladaptive behaviour' (for example, perseveration) and 'functional activities' (for example, sweeping the floor). The nurse can build up a systematic picture of a client from using schedules such as the *BOI*, providing a basis for the care plan (for example, the evaluation phase). Other schedules do not specify any behaviours in advance, but ask the nurse to note whatever a client is doing at certain intervals (time sampling) or to record every time a behaviour of interest occurs (event sampling).

Which technique is best?

The answer to this question echoes that offered to earlier ones: consider the details of each case in relation to the available options. In order to do this, the nurse has to have a good working knowledge of the options, or access to someone with this knowledge. Psychologists are usually able to help with the selection of an appropriate technique, or the nurse can consult a resource book of suitable instruments. In either case it will probably be necessary to try out (pilot) a technique in order to assess its suitability. The details of a particular client or context may alter the value or appropriateness of a given technique, so it is best to adopt a scientific approach and test out instruments in the situation in which they are to be used. Reliability is one such scientific consideration (see Chapter 3), where you should check that your observations agree with those made independently by your colleagues.

There are also some practical criteria by which to judge an instrument, including how long it takes to complete an assessment, and how difficult it is to apply in a precise fashion. For these reasons some instruments, such as intelligence and personality tests, are unsuitable for nursing administration: such instruments are used by psychologists only after extensive training. However, even these relatively sophisticated tools can suffer from major practical drawbacks, leading to the need to weigh up the benefits of a particular instrument against the cost of applying it. (I will return to the strengths and weaknesses of the different assessment methods in the final section of this chapter.)

A case study

Jean was a 29-year-old mother of two who was referred to the Community Psychiatric Nursing (CPN) Service by her GP because of anxiety. She had recently moved to the area and had lost the support of friends she had made whilst living in the Midlands. Also, her family were in Ireland, so she had little contact with them. She presented with acute anxiety about her husband's work commitments and the resulting lack of support and contact with him too. There had been some disagreement between them about her looking for work, his feelings being that her priorities lay with their two children and that she should be content with the role of mother.

In essence, Jean seemed lonely, unsupported and unable to develop herself as a person. Additionally, the differences between the couple had been highlighted by the move up North. Her low self-esteem made her inclined to blame herself for the current situation, and it took two sessions of individual work before she would accept that there was a need for conjoint work.

In terms of our main headings, the CPN involved was employing the following assessment methods:

Assessment strategies and instruments

A semi-structured interview format and observation represented the two main strategies. The interview was based on *life stages*, that is, a view in which life events and the related transitions are treated as particularly significant, following the work of Brown and Harris (1978) and family therapists such as Burnham (1986).

Figure 4.3 summarises the interview structure. The symbols indicate the different life events which are likely to occur at each of the seven identified life stages. For example, in Jean's case the stage 'maturity to middle age' would be expected to be associated with 'familial/interactional' difficulties. The CPN therefore knew that these were probably worth discussing with Jean, and this turned out to be the case. However, the nurse routinely considers life events in relation to all four aspects of the client's functioning.

The observations of Jean and her husband were based on video tape recordings. He started to participate after the first two inter-views. The CPN watched these recordings following sessions, in the company of her supervision team. Together they reviewed what had happened and reconsidered 'the problem' and how to address it. In essence, this involved generating hypotheses about the couple which might explain Jean's anxiety. The CPN then tested these hypotheses out in the next session, or after a 'time-out' period during the session.

In addition to the structured interview and video tape recordings, the CPN occasionally uses such assessment techniques as 'sculpting' (a family therapy technique, based on asking clients to physically position the other family members in such a way as to indicate their perceived relationships), diaries, family trees, questionnaires, and 'enactment' (where the clients are asked to re-enact a relevant scene, such as their discussion about therapy, for the therapist during the interview stage). The most common approach, however, is to encourage the family to discuss a problematic issue.

Who collects the information?

As indicated already, in Jean's case the information was gathered primarily by the therapist, but also by the supervision team (usually 2–3 nurses with a special interest in family therapy) and by the couple themselves. In other cases the CPN may seek comments from significant others, such as members of the extended family or friends.

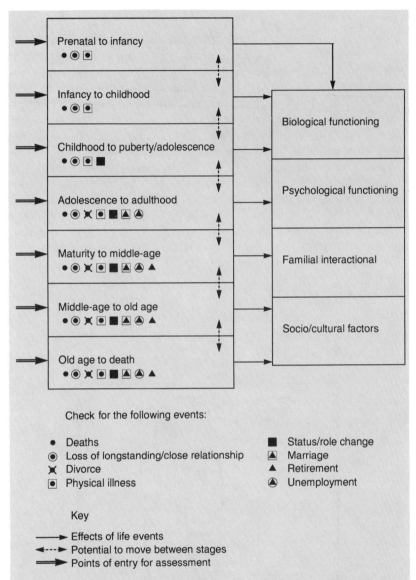

Check for the following events:

- Deaths
- Loss of longstanding/close relationship
- Divorce
- Physical illness

- Status/role change
- Marriage
- Retirement
- Unemployment

Key

→ Effects of life events
◄--► Potential to move between stages
⇒ Points of entry for assessment

Figure 4.4 *The CPN's structured interview for major life events.*

Where is the information gathered?

Initially Jean was seen in her own home by the CPN. After a couple of appointments they moved to a project centre in the local high street. This was an accessible and non-stigmatised venue, complete with the audio-visual equipment mentioned earlier.

When are assessments made?

This refers to the point in time when the clients are seen and to the sequencing of the assessment methods. In the nurse's opinion there was a clear reason for Jean's referral. This was her move to the North East, associated with a loss of her support network and her great difficulty in establishing new relationships. Jean turned to her husband for extra support to compensate, but he continued to work very long hours and attributed her difficulties entirely to herself ('it's your problem'), thus avoiding a supportive role.

Jean and her husband have been seen weekly or fortnightly by the CPN, who started the assessment process by interviewing Jean alone, moving on to the use of video recordings after a couple of sessions (that is, after two hours or so). However, as stressed in Chapter 3, the nurse repeatedly returns to assessment questions and methods throughout therapy. This indicates how inseparable assessment and therapy can be in some models.

What to assess?

The problem was phrased very generally by the referring GP, alluding only to Jean's anxiety state. As far as this side of the

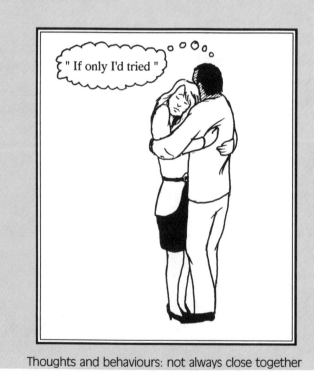

Thoughts and behaviours: not always close together

'problem' was concerned, the CPN defined the anxiety in terms of the triple response system of thoughts, feelings and behaviours. Thoughts included self-depreciation (for example, 'I've never achieved anything'; 'I'm not intelligent enough to mix') and a fear of being judged negatively by others. Prominent feelings were a churning stomach and feeling hot and sweaty. Key behaviours were talking quickly, difficulty in taking her children to school, avoiding other mums when there and also avoiding as far as possible trips to the shops and similar places.

However, the nurse also wanted to define the problem in terms of Jean's marital relationship. Here a major difficulty lay in their poor communication patterns and what she referred to as 'inadequate intimacy'. This meant that Jean and husband were not allowing or encouraging each other to develop, but were rather 'tramlining' one another into stereotyped roles as 'breadwinner' (husband works 12-hour days and also part of the weekends) and 'childcarer'. They were therefore locked like tramwheels into a 'parallel working' relationship in which they never really met or developed, and which maintained Jean's anxiety in a pathological relationship pattern. By viewing the presenting problem (Jean's anxiety) in this way, the nurse felt able to understand what was going on and to decide how best to intervene (in this case by working with the couple).

Strengths and weaknesses of assessment methods

There is no single assessment method which is always to be preferred, regardless of the circumstances. Equally, there are other methods which will rarely seem appropriate, given a particular assessment model. For instance, it is rare for psychodynamic therapists to use questionnaires and common for family therapists to employ direct observation. Allowing for these general assessment strategies, within any one model there is a need to use methods sensitively and flexibly. Some clients will be upset on reading a long list of their symptoms on a questionnaire, others hugely relieved ('I'm not alone'). Some clients are able to maintain accurate and informative diaries, while others are so disorganised or apathetic that just attending an appointment is an achievement. Given such individual differences in clients and therapists, what general points can be made about the assessment methods? Three criteria have been used to address this question.

How practical is the assessment instrument?

Any assessment method has to be considered in terms of such basic questions as how difficult it is to apply or how long it takes to complete. There is little value in having a very comprehensive assessment instrument which takes so long to complete that it is rarely used. Similarly, we might favour those instruments which provide clear and readily interpreted results. Some methods, such as the psychodynamic therapist's assessment of dreams, require extensive training and considerable judgement. Others, such as Baker and Hall's *REHAB* (1983) provide a relatively quick and clear result.

Exercise 4.1: Judging an assessment instrument

A list of such practical factors is given in *Table 4.2*. This is based on Anastasi's work (1976). As an exercise, try addressing these factors in relation to an assessment instrument. You can find examples of assessment instruments in scientific journals: Chambless *et al.* (1985) produced a questionnaire for assessing agoraphobia, Vrana *et al.* (1986) developed a structured interview for assessing dental fear, Davidson and Raistrick (1986) offered a questionnaire on alcohol dependence, while Baker (1985; pp134–153) provided a system for rating a wide range of behaviours seen in psychiatric in-patients. Examples of this kind of analysis of assessment instruments can be found in McDowell and Newell (1987), and Peck and Shapiro (1991).

Table 4.2 *A list of some of the practical factors to be considered in selecting an assessment instrument*

Factors	Practical issues
1. Administration	How easy is it to use? Is extensive training required?
2. Appropriateness	Is it relevant to your clients? (for example, language differences)
3. Time	How long does it take to administer?
4. Availability	Can you obtain the instrument, together with any manual? Can you afford it?
5. Clarity	Are the directions for using it clear?
6. Scoring	Is it clear how the clients' replies are to be scored or analysed? Is this straightforward or time-consuming?
7. Interpretation	How is information to be interpreted or understood?
8. Rapport	Will the instrument put clients off, or can it help to improve the therapist/client relationship?

What are the 'technical' standards of the assessment instruments'?

If an assessment device has been published in a scientific journal it is very probably a sound instrument. This is to say that it has been considered in terms of its reliability, validity and, if appropriate, its norms. If the device had been found seriously wanting in one of these regards it would not have been published. Publishing therefore provides something of a vetting service, and an instrument found in a scientific journal is probably far more sound technically than the kinds of instruments that tend to be found in office filing cabinets and which have an unknown origin. These usually lack any technical data and may never have been vetted (see Hall (1979) for a review and discussion). As a consequence they may be like the 'elastic ruler' discussed in Chapter 3, giving unreliable or invalid measurements. To remind you, *reliability* refers to how consistently an instrument measures whatever it is intended to measure, while *validity* concerns the extent to which an instrument actually does measure what it is intended to measure. *Norms*, the third technical criterion mentioned above, are the figures which authors provide indicating how defined groups of people have scored on a particular instrument. This offers a comparison point for any score obtained with an individual client.

How useful is an assessment instrument?

We can conceive of a measure which is highly 'practical' and 'technically' sound, yet which is of little relevance. It may tell us nothing of value concerning the formulation of a client's problem, nor indicate how to proceed with therapy, nor indeed provide any useful measure of the outcome of therapy. For this reason *utility* is often added to the criteria for judging an instrument. Utility is usually defined as the degree to which a tool contributes to assessment and therapy (Hayes *et al.*, 1987).

Clinical psychologists are keenly aware of this criterion, as for many years they were routinely asked by psychiatrists to provide I.Q. and personality assessments of clients. It was rarely clear what these time-consuming but technically sound assessments contributed to their clients' care. For this and other reasons psychologists have moved away from routine assessments.

What are the general strengths and weaknesses of the different methods?

Assessment instruments can vary in terms of their practical and technical characteristics, and in their utility. These considerations are true of all methods, and should be borne in mind when selecting an instrument. In addition to these three considerations there are some general strengths and weaknesses with all methods. There is no simple answer to the question 'which one is 'best'?' I will therefore consider the strengths and weaknesses of the main methods, so that you can decide which to use for each specific task.

Interview

This most time-honoured and popular form of assessment has much to recommend it, including the opportunity to hear about a problem directly from a client (or significant others) and the chance to seek clarification and generally to relate the interview to the client and the problem. It therefore has considerable utility and flexibility, and tends to appeal to both therapist and client.

On the debit side, it is relatively time-consuming when the therapist's aim is to gather lots of information quickly (questionnaires or diary record sheets, for instance, are a much quicker option). Reliability and validity can be highly suspect, as the interview is based on the client's self-report and is often conducted in the context of considerable emotional arousal (for example, anger or fear). The therapist may also introduce bias by selectively attending to easy or favoured topics, at the expense of a comprehensive assessment. For example, it is tempting to try and arrive at a quick and clear formulation of a problem so as to fulfil one's therapeutic role, and this pressure can be communicated in subtle ways to the client who then colludes in order to fulfil their role as a motivated client. Since this can be such a subtle process, and as there is often no other information to go on, both therapist and client can be significantly misled. One is struck by this when comparing notes with another person who has seen the same client but who presents a rather different picture. The structured interview can reduce many of these inherent weaknesses and offer a valuable adjunct to other measures.

Self-ratings

Such instruments as clinical diaries, rating scales, questionnaires and record sheets do afford the kind of structure which is often missing in interviews, and they can help the client to generate a great deal of information in a short period of time. Indeed, as this is often the client's own time, the savings in time and effort can be considerable. If these self-report (sometimes also referred to as 'paper and pencil') measures are drawn from the scientific journals, there is also the possibility of relating your client to other 'known' groups by looking at the norms. Particularly in the case of symptomatic questionnaires, you can be more confident about a problem's definition or severity by considering norms. It is also easy to repeat the measure in order to evaluate your care plan.

Questionnaires evoke mixed reaction from clinicians, some fearing, for instance, that they will offend or upset clients. In my experience, the reverse is more often the case, as when a client can see from the questions on the form that they are not the only person in the world with certain difficulties (the sometimes powerful phenomenon of *universality*). Some forms can also help the client to see new ways of coping, or to understand their problem better. For example, I have sent my out-patients questionnaires addressing their stress, coping and strain before the first appointment and these encouraged some of them to reconsider their problem from this perspective (for example, 'maybe I'm not going mad; maybe I'm just experiencing a lot of stress for which my coping strategies are inadequate').

Record sheets, diaries and self-ratings are more commonly used to help to formulate the problem or to monitor progress. They tend to require more of the client than the interview does (for example, literacy and motivation) and so may often not be completed or fail to furnish useful information. However, sometimes these 'compliance' difficulties can also afford a therapeutic opportunity, as in helping a client to become more expert at self-monitoring, or in achieving objectives.

The weakest aspect of self-rating is perhaps the reliance on what the client is able to report, and this has many pitfalls. The reliability and validity questions loom as large as they do for the interview, but in the case of self-ratings there may also be little or no utility. Again, carefully developed and properly organised methods, such as questionnaires, can minimise these difficulties.

The other major objections are perhaps the ones concerning the impersonal and general nature of self-ratings. There may be an implication that clients are not being treated humanely as individuals, which will run counter to the message therapists wish to convey. The lack of time and effort they invest in self-ratings may similarly undermine the therapeutic alliance, particularly when the therapist only gives the client's material a cursory glance and does not integrate it with the care plan.

Direct observation

This method scores most highly on validity. Observation also usually implies very focused attention on behaviour in relation to a few key situations. This can help us to understand problems in ways that interviews and self-ratings cannot. And of course some clients cannot (or will not) comply with other assessment methods, making observation the main option.

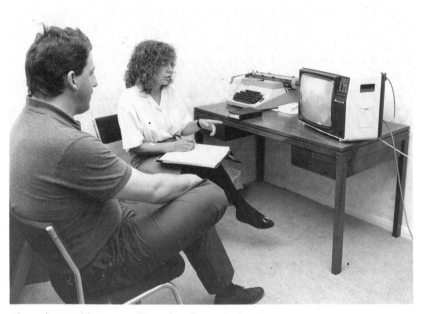

Observing a video recording of a client's behaviour

Observation is often time consuming, if not because of the actual time spent recording then because the therapist has to observe in situations where the problem arises. With out-patients this can mean home visits or trips to work or the town centre. This effort can be repaid by the high utility of the information: often observation will reveal important insights into problems that even highly verbal clients cannot disclose. Reliability, however, is a problem and care needs to be taken that two or more nurses are observing in a similar fashion with the same results.

Summary

I have suggested that there is no one 'best' method of assessing clients' problems. All strategies and instruments have their strengths and weaknesses, so the best approach is to weigh these up in relation to the client concerned and the kind of information you require. In general, it is a good idea to combine methods, for example, using interviews to get an overview of the problem, then using questionnaires to elicit more detailed information. By combining methods in this way we also tend to improve the validity and utility of our assessment, two major obstacles in assessment. The two other obstacles identified were reliability and the practical aspects of an assessment (such as the time or training it takes to apply it).

Questions for further consideration

1 In relation to the 'assessment grid' (*Figure 4.1*), where would you place the following?
   a) an observational scale, such as the *Behaviour Observation Instrument*
   b) a biofeedback machine which measures skin conductance (moistness of the skin)
   c) a client's 'diary record' of their negative thoughts about themselves.
2 On the same theme of classifying different assessment instruments, how would you distinguish between a nurse's rating scale for assessing client mood and a 'social activities' questionnaire completed by clients?
3 Try to list a range of situations in which a client's self-report goes from being highly appropriate to being minimally valuable (for example, in relation to a diagnosis or the type of self-report instrument).
4 How might you assess a client's thoughts, feelings and behaviours when the problems are:
   a) an obsessional-compulsive disorder?
   b) schizophrenia?
   c) depression?
5 Why do we do the things we do? Attempt to formulate (analyse) one of your own behaviours in relation to a model of your own choice (for example, smoking; a hobby).
6 In discussion with nursing staff on a local psychiatric ward, see if you can tease out a range of problem formulations for the clients on the ward.
7 Under what circumstances would direct observation be the assessment strategy of choice?
8 Which assessment instruments would you add to those listed in this chapter? Why?

References

Alevizos, P., Derisi, W., Liberman, R., Eckman, T. and Callahan, E. (1978). The *Behaviour Observation Instrument*: a method for direct observation for programme evaluation. *Journal of Applied Behaviour Analysis, 11*, 243–257.
Anastasi, A. (1976). *Psychological Testing*. Collier-Macmillan, London.
Baker, R. D. and Hall, J. N. (1983). *REHAB: A Rehabilitation Evaluation Rating Scale*. Aberdeen: Vine Publishing.

Barker, P. J. (1985). *Patient Assessment in Psychiatric Nursing.* London: Croom Helm.

Beck, A. T., Ward, C. H., Mendleson, M., Mock, J. and Erbaugh, J. (1961). An inventory for measuring depression. *Archives of General Psychiatry, 4*, 53–63.

Brown, G. and Harris, T. (1978). *Social Origins of Depression: A Study of Psychiatric Disorder in Women.* London: Tavistock.

Burnham, J. (1986). *Family Therapy.* London: Tavistock.

Carnwath, T. and Miller, D. (1986). *Behavioural Psychotherapy in Primary Care.* London: Academic Press.

Chambless, D. L., Cauputo, G. C., Jasin, S. E., Gracely, E. J. and Williams, C. (1985). The Mobility Inventory for Agoraphobia. *Behaviour Research and Therapy, 23*, 35–44.

Cone, J. D. (1978). The Behavioural Assessment Grid (BAG): a conceptual framework and taxonomy. *Behaviour Therapy, 9*, 882–888.

Davidson, R. J. and Raistrick, D. (1986). The validity of the Short Alcohol Dependence Data (SADD) Questionnaire. *British Journal of Addiction, 81*, 217–222.

Hall, J. N. (1979). Assessment procedures used in studies on long-stay patients. *British Journal of Psychiatry, 135*, 330–335.

Hayes, S. C., Nelson, R. O. and Jarrett, R. B. (1987). The treatment utility of assessment. *American Psychologist, 42*, 963–974.

Honigfeld, G. (1966). *Nurses Observation Scale for Inpatient Evaluation (NOSIE-30).* Glen Oaks, New York: Honigfeld.

Kingston, B. (1987). *Psychological Approaches in Psychiatric Nursing.* London: Croom Helm.

Marks, I. M., Hallam, R. S., Connolly, J. and Philpotts, R. (1977). *Nursing in behavioural psychotherapy.* London: Royal College of Nursing.

Marks, I. M. (1985). *Psychiatric Nurse Therapists in Primary Care.* London: Royal College of Nursing.

McDowell, I. and Newell, C. (1987). *Measuring Health: A Guide to Rating Scales and Questionnaires.* Oxford: Oxford University Press.

Pattie, A. H. and Gilleard, C. J. (1979). *Manual of the Clifton Assessment Procedures for the Elderly (CAPE).* Kent: Hodder and Stoughton.

Peck, D. and Shapiro, C. (1991). *Measuring Human Problems: A Practical Guide.* Chichester: Wiley.

Platt, S., Weyman, A., Hirsch, S. and Hewett, S. (1980). The *Social Behaviour Assessment Schedule (SBAS)*: rationale, contents, scoring and reliability, of a new interview schedule. *Social Psychiatry, 15*, 43–55.

Rachman, S. (1978). *Fear and Courage.* San Francisco: Freeman.

Vrana, S., McNeil, D. W. and McGlynn, F. D. (1986). A structured interview for assessing dental fear. *Journal of Behaviour Therapy and Experimental Psychiatry, 17*, 175–178.

Wing, J. K. (1961). A simple and reliable subclassification of chronic schizophrenia. *Journal of Mental Science, 107*, 862–875.

Woods, R. T. and Britton, P. G. (1985). *Clinical Psychology with the Elderly.* London: Routledge.

Further reading

Anastasi, A. (1976). *Psychological Testing.* London: Macmillan.
    This is one of the classics on assessment and covers all the main issues such as reliability and validity.

West, J. and Spinks, P. (1988). *Clinical Psychology in Action.* London: Wright.

A rare view of what psychologists do in their diverse activities, presented in the form of brief, readable case studies. Each one has an assessment section, and these provide many interesting ideas.

Nelson, R. O. and Hayes, S. C. (Eds; 1986). *Conceptual Foundations of Behavioural Assessment*. London: Guilford Press.
Nelson and Hayes provide a radical rethink of assessment from a behavioural model.

Barker, P. J. (1985). *Patient Assessment in Psychiatric Nursing*. London: Croom Helm.
Dr Barker considers methods for the assessment of anxiety, depression, relationship, psychosis and everyday living skills.

SECTION THREE

Planning

5 _Planning tasks_

The information gathered in the assessment phase of the nursing process is used to try and make sense of the client's problem, prior to commencing therapy. This phase, termed _problem analysis_, represents a bridge between assessment and therapy. If the assessment has been successful, then the nurse is in a position to understand the problem and move forward. From this base, decisions can be made about an intervention. Indeed, such is the importance of problem analysis that it can also serve as therapy, as the client's bewilderment and worst fears can be eased by a plausible account of the problem.

Despite its crucial role, problem analysis is strikingly absent from most published care plans (for example, Marks, 1986). To redress the balance, I will spend some time outlining some of the analyses which have been provided in mental health. These will encompass the main therapeutic models.

I will then look at the choice of therapeutic objectives, or 'goals' as I will refer to them. Having explained a problem, the nurse considers the available options in relation to the possible goals. Basically, the question to be addressed is: how can we get from here (the problem) to there (the solution)? Difficulties can arise as readily from overambitious goal-setting as from the more commonly blamed therapeutic techniques. And again, the very act of clarifying small achievable goals can contribute in a significant way to therapy.

Another crossroads encountered in this chapter is that between goals and evaluation. As evaluation concerns the extent to which goals are achieved, clearly the two are interdependent. Although the evaluation of our therapeutic services is increasingly requested by managers and others, few of these services actually have the kind of goals that permit evaluation (Milne, 1987). The most common statement of objectives is usually more like a general philosophy of care than a list of realisable goals. This state of affairs partly reflects the difficulty in clarifying goals in what are often complex systems; thankfully goal-setting in therapeutic activities is more straightforward.

The final aim of this chapter is to demonstrate these points in the form of a case study. I will again draw this from the routine work of mental health nurses from a typical large institution in the North East of England. This time I will consider the problem of depression in the context of an acute ward.

Analysis: making sense of clinical problems

Once assessment information has been gathered, the next task is to use
it to understand the client. This understanding paves the way to the
selection and success of an intervention.

Problem analysis (also known as *formulation*) refers to the everyday
phenomenon of trying to describe and explain things. But while it is
the stuff of casual conversations, it is also the major task of scientific
enquiry. Reading my Sunday paper before I set to work on this
chapter, I was struck by a rather good example of problem analysis
spanning conversation and science. The headline read: 'Sunbathing
reduces the risk of breast cancer'. Written by the newspaper's science
correspondent, the article reported the findings of a team of scientists
in New Orleans. By studying the frequency of breast cancer in relation
to average amounts of sunlight in the USA, Russia and Japan, these
researchers concluded that exposure to sunlight acted as a deterrent to
breast cancer. So far this describes a relationship between one thing
and another: cancer was three times as frequent in those Russian
republics with relatively low sunshine levels, for instance. The
researchers were also able to go one step further than this correlational
statement to explain their findings. It seemed that the sunlight was a
causal agent in that it triggered the natural production of Vitamin D, a
substance understood to protect against cancer, apparently by encouraging cells to bind together more effectively and so to regulate each
other's growth. Evidence for this came from the Japanese sample,
which had the lowest levels of cancer. It seemed that their diet,
exceptionally high in Vitamin D, complemented the effect of sunlight
on the body's own production of Vitamin D. Those Japanese who went
to live in the USA or UK and altered their diets suffered slowly
increasing rates of the cancer.

In this fascinating article (McKie, 1990) one can see both problem
description and explanation, with the explanation taking the form of a
specific causal agent (Vitamin D). This is exactly the kind of logic that
one is seeking in problem analysis, although the causal agents in
mental health are usually rather different. However, as in this
example, the concern is to try to use assessment information to guide
the intervention. In the article the obvious therapy was Vitamin D, but
this was not immediately obvious from the description of an association
between sunlight and cancer. The researchers 'discovered' the significance of Vitamin D because their medical model guided them towards
the most likely explanation. They knew what sort of thing they were
looking for and where to find it. When they found it, they knew how
to make sense of it.

This example rather neatly illustrates the main issue in problem analysis, namely that of problem description and problem explanation. These are to be attempted in such a way that they are consistent with a given model, and so suggest the best form of therapy. I have already considered how best to define and describe a problem in Chapter 4, so the focus here is on the link between explanation and therapy. Suffice to say that the model which guided problem description should also guide the other stages of the nursing process. This should be clear from what I said about models in Chapter 1, that is, that a conceptual model colours how we look at things, whether in assessment or therapy. The illustrations that follow will hopefully underline this point, while indicating how problems can be analysed in routine clinical practice.

In very general terms, each therapeutic approach carries with it some major assumptions about causes and cures. Psychiatry tends to be associated with a biological model in which things like brain damage or biochemical disorders are regarded as paramount. In contrast, psychodynamically-orientated psychotherapists would be expected to consider unconscious processes as the most significant phenomena. At a more detailed level, the therapeutic models may suggest some of the specific mechanisms which are thought to explain the problem. For instance, in the case of depression the psychoanalyst will be particularly alert for signs that the client has internalised the hostility they felt when they lost someone for whom they had mixed feelings; or for signs that the client is reacting to their separation from something or somebody of particular significance. However, these explanations are still rather general, attempting as they do to include all clients with depression (or whatever the problem might be). As striking illustrations of this kind of general explanation, consider the following statements from a book of case studies by an assistant of Freud's, Wilhelm Stekel (1923):

> We realise what severe psychic conflicts these unfortunate patients inwardly struggle against. It is, as a matter of fact, always virtue that makes them neurotic (p194).

> The majority of neuroses owe their development to unhappy marriages (p218).

> In no phobia may we forget the never-failing criminal basis (p319).

Although obviously an old book, the tendency to this kind of general explanation is ever present in all therapy models, since, as Stekel points out 'one need only have one's eyes open, then it will not be possible to overlook these things' (p155). We might add that what one sees is determined by the particular model which has opened one's eyes, rather than being some kind of obvious fact. A behavioural psychotherapist, to take but one example, would probably be quite blind to the role of a 'criminal basis' in the case of a phobia.

Let me now proceed to the level of problem analysis of individual cases. These draw on the more general levels of analysis already mentioned, but proceed to a more detailed and specific explanation.

Examples of problem analysis

Cognitive therapy

A 40-year-old mother of two with long-standing depression (including 8 years on medication) presented with low self-esteem, obsessional regard over her appearance, apprehension about coping once her children left home, and a pessimistic view of the future. In general, she perceived herself as a burden on her husband, and an inadequate mother.

Assessment indicated that her depressed moods were associated with negative thoughts about her worth as a person, such as 'I'm a hopeless wife. He's better off without me' These thoughts were usually triggered off by social encounters when she felt 'put down' or inadequate in some way. Feelings of despair and emotional withdrawal followed, resulting in a reduction in her effectiveness as a mother and wife. As a response to her obvious difficulties, her husband would try to help out, but she saw this as further evidence of her worthlessness. Also, the assessment indicated that the husband misperceived his wife's withdrawal as a sign of lack of caring towards him. This often led to his making cutting remarks, which then set off another cycle of self-depreciation in his wife. *Figure 5.1* illustrates this process.

The depression was therefore analysed in terms of the wife's irrational beliefs, which served to maintain her low self-esteem and to draw her husband into a cycle of mutual destruction. The associated feelings included anger, distress, passive aggression and depression. As this was an example of 'cognitive therapy' (from West and Spinks, 1988) it is appropriate to find that the problem is understood in terms of faulty thinking patterns. In particular, the therapist was able to point out how the couple had consistently misinterpreted each other's behaviour, and to highlight a fundamental irrational belief. This was that after 20 years of marriage, a couple should be able to read each other's minds. The therapist helped both partners to acknowledge their share of responsibility for more effective communication, and so reduced the inappropriate perceptions each had developed towards the other's behaviour. They were encouraged to develop ways of challenging these perceptions, in order to be able to alter their feelings and behaviour.

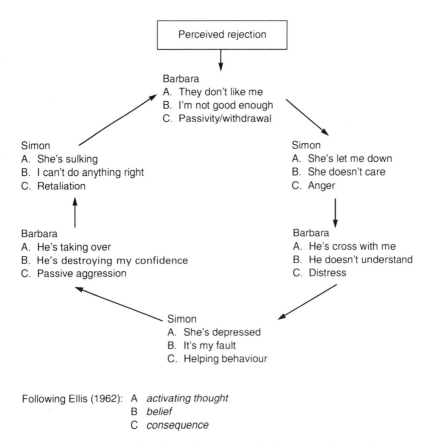

Following Ellis (1962): A *activating thought*
                          B *belief*
                          C *consequence*

Figure 5.1 *An example of problem analysis in depression, using a cognitive therapy approach. (Reproduced from West and Spinks (1988) by permission of Butterworth Scientific Ltd.)*

Behaviour therapy

A similar causal chain of events is presumed to explain problems from a behavioural standpoint. Again, it is assumed that problems do not emerge without good cause, but in behaviour therapy this cause is to be found in what we do. That is, while clients may complain of problems with their thoughts or feelings, the behaviour therapist expects to be able to resolve these by concentrating therapy on some form of inappropriate or maladaptive behaviour. In essence, the thoughts and feelings are seen as real and important, but as secondary to what the client is doing or not doing.

The assessment concerns events which are going on around the client, and in which the client is in some way involved. The therapist will therefore seek information on stressful events, such as relationship difficulties or facing up to a feared object. In the case of an obsessional-compulsive disorder, the client may be distressed at discovering a film of dust on top of the furniture, or on seeing a member of the family bringing some dirt into the house. This may lead to high levels of anxiety, which the client may try to reduce by a 'ritual', such as repeated hand-washing or cleaning. As a consequence the client may experience relief from the anxiety, perhaps thinking that the house is now 'clean' and feeling relieved at this.

The behavioural analysis is therefore based on antecedent events (such as dirt, dust) that stress the individual and trigger off behaviours (for example, washing and cleaning rituals) which in turn serve to reduce the stressor and any associated thoughts and feelings. The essential reason for such problems is regarded as faulty learning, in the sense that a client can develop, through repeated conditioning experiences, a set of responses which only affords a temporary solution. To return to the example of a compulsive ritual, by providing relief the washing or cleaning behaviours are 'reinforced'. This means that they are even more likely to happen the next time the client is stressed by dirt or dust.

In some cases, the kind of conditioning that occurs is primarily of the 'classical' kind, that is, a client learns to respond to a stimulus. In other instances the process of 'operant conditioning' is paramount: this is when a client's behaviour can be understood to be affecting their environment. Behaviour therapists also recognise that maladaptive behaviour can be learnt by observing what other people do ('modelling') or by information (for example, reading) and that in any one case there is typically a mixture of learning processes at work (Rachman, 1977).

Psychodynamic therapy

In cognitive or behaviour therapy the focus is on distressing thoughts or behaviours which are known to the client, and which are assumed to be 'the problem'. Psychodynamic therapy, by comparison, considers that symptoms, such as washing rituals, have an unconscious basis. The therapist's task is to bring the unconscious basis for the symptoms to the client's awareness, termed 'insight'.

Kingston (1987) has provided an example of a psychodynamic formulation for an obsessional-compulsive disorder. She cited the case of a 29-year-old woman who engaged in cleaning rituals, in particular excessive washing in relation to her 6-month-old baby (for example, showering before each feeding of her baby and washing her hands four times after she changed her).

The assessment indicated that the client had been separated from her father almost from birth, and that her mother had maintained a negative picture of the father. The client and her mother had grown up in a very close relationship, to the extent that they saw each other as near perfect. Their harmony continued when the client married, but through therapy it became clear that she felt intensively ambivalent about her mother, on one hand loving and needing her, on the other rejecting and hating her. Such was their relationship that she felt unable to express her feelings of being trapped and angry, and instead made every effort to please her mother. With the birth of her own baby, the client began to realise that she longed for her father and felt a sense of loss about her relationship with him. She saw her mother as the reason for this loss and so began to feel angry and resentful towards her. The client also came to feel intensely resentful towards her baby, as she regarded the baby as better cared for than she had been.

The client in this case study had some awareness of these thoughts and feelings, but was unconscious of the real reasons for them, or for her compulsive rituals. The psychodynamic analysis was that the rituals served as a defence against her anxieties about harming the baby, as a result of her strong feelings of resentment towards the baby. The excessive care and cleanliness served to deny the underlying feelings she had towards her child. Just as with her own relationship with her mother, no suggestion of hostility or rejection was allowed. However, this defence mechanism became too much of a burden to bear, and so the client entered therapy. During the process of therapy she became more aware of what motivated her rituals, helped by the therapeutic alliance and the therapist's use of interpretation and other psychodynamic techniques.

Client-centred counselling

Insight in psychodynamic therapy is an extreme kind of self-awareness. Other therapists also value insight, but they tend not to see it as the necessary and sufficient basis for cure. Thus, cognitive and behaviour therapists may ask their clients to study videos or keep diaries in order to improve their understanding of themselves. But this is in a straightforwardly educational sense, and can be compared to helping a man with a sexual dysfunction realise that the reason for his difficulty is partly beyond his voluntary control – he can't simply will himself to have an erection.

The *non-directive* or *client-centred* approach to therapy lies somewhere between the psychodynamic and the behavioural models with regard to self-awareness. Loosely referred to as *counselling*, these approaches derive from a humanistic theory in which the client's inner experience and self-fulfilment are primary. The counsellor's task is to help the client understand him or herself better through a range of verbal relationship techniques, such as clarifying what the client is saying or delineating therapy goals.

Consider the following case study in counselling, provided by Hokanson (1983). A young man with a history of delinquency and anti-social behaviour is being seen by the counsellor. This client behaves in a suspicious manner, as if expecting rejection at any stage. He seems detached and angry, engaging in provocative acts which appear to be intended to secure a negative reaction from the therapist. The therapist responds by trying to make sense of the client's predicament and by recognising the provocations, but steadfastly refusing to be drawn into a negative response. Instead, support and friendship are offered consistently by the counsellor.

The therapist is helped to react in this remarkably controlled and sympathetic way by the analysis of the client's problem. The provocation and anger, for instance, are not perceived by counselling therapists as being directed at them in any meaningful sense. Rather, they would be inclined to understand that clients such as this one have experienced traumatic childhoods, often centred on failed relationships. In Hokanson's case study (1983, pp200–2), the young man never appeared to have established a predictable and deep relationship with either of his parents. Loneliness and fear seemed to dominate his early life, as he was neglected or unacknowledged by his parents. In part, this was related to his own demands for attention, which became increasingly loud and inappropriate. A spiral of mutual aversive control developed in the family, so that when he demanded attention

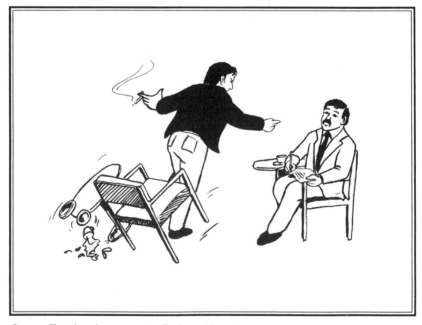

Counselling involves a controlled reaction to anger

his parents would often beat him in a sustained and violent manner. The spiral worsened as he thought of new ways to get back at his parents. This kind of pattern had persisted through school until the time of therapy.

Viewing the client in terms of this sort of personal history can make it much easier for the therapist to offer help. In addition, the counselling therapist may make sense of clients in relation to such concepts as the denial of inner experience, alienation from oneself and an absence of meaning in life. For example, in the case given here, the client would dismiss his father's eventual departure from the household with the comment 'It really didn't matter' and by expressing no interest in himself or the future.

The value of problem analysis

These analyses provide therapists with some vital ingredients for therapy. They help to describe and explain the problem, which gives therapy the necessary direction. They also help to explain the problem from the perspective of each individual client, as opposed to a diagnosis which so often leads to a fairly uniform treatment. Lastly, problem analysis helps therapists to do a good job, by enabling them to distinguish between the client's feelings for them and for others. They therefore do not have to relate to clients as most other people do, thus setting the scene for effective therapy.

While the details of these therapeutic models differ quite noticeably, the essential elements of a psychological analysis can be seen in all of them. As illustrated in *Figure 5.2* and discussed in Chapter 1, these are some form of 'stressor'; possibly some sensitivity or 'vulnerability' which makes the stress particularly telling (such as irrational beliefs); the presence of conscious or unconscious forms of 'coping'; and the result of unsuccessful coping, seen in the form of 'strain'. When someone copes directly with stress they feel good about themselves, experiencing what is referred to as *mastery*. When the coping is less direct, then 'getting by' might be a better expression.

Exercise 5.1: A stress–coping–strain analysis
As an exercise, try to analyse a client's problem using this general 'stress–coping–strain' approach. A practical way to arrange this is to have one person role-play a client they know well. The group conducts an interview of this 'client', each person in the group asking the questions which they see as important for this kind of assessment and analysis. These could include: What makes the problem worse? How can the problem be eased? Can you describe the distress you experience? At the end of the role-play you should try to produce a problem analysis.

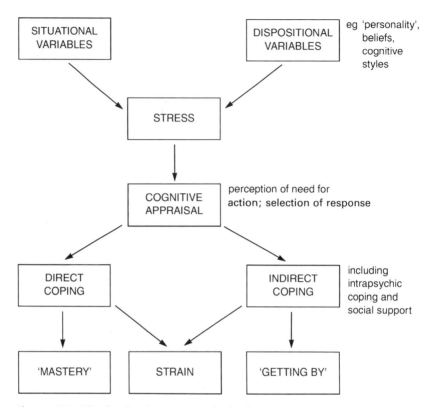

Figure 5.2 *The basis of most psychological analyses of problem (after Lazarus, 1974).*

Goal-setting: establishing therapeutic objectives

Why set goals?

In the preceding case studies I glossed over the step between analysis and therapy. For some therapies this gloss is quite real, in that the therapist will not see it as appropriate to spend time clarifying goals with the clients. But they will still have some objectives in mind, at least for themselves. To illustrate, most therapists will aim to get a clear picture of the problem, build up a therapeutic alliance and to analyse, intervene and evaluate. Also, even if not discussed with the client, therapists have some form of ending in mind as a general goal.

However, cognitive, behavioural and counselling therapies, together with most others, will work on goals in a deliberate and detailed way, in full collaboration with the client. This is because goals are seen as a necessary part of therapy, and client participation in setting goals is regarded as extremely important. When it is not possible for the client to participate in goal-setting, then the nurse still needs to determine what is being attempted. One example is the selection of goals for elderly people who are too disorientated to enter into goal-setting. Barrowclough and Fleming (1986) have developed a manual designed for this purpose, and this provides a clear illustration of goal-setting.

Why bother to set goals? On a purely logical note, it is not possible to evaluate your care plan if there are no goals, since 'evaluation' is defined as the extent to which goals are achieved. (More on this in Chapters 7 and 8.) On practical grounds, goals serve a number of useful functions. In a review of research, Locke *et al.* (1981) stated that: 'Goals affect performance by directing attention, mobilising effort, increasing persistence and motivating strategy development' (p125). Defining 'goals' as what an individual is trying to accomplish, they found that specific and optimally difficult ('challenging') goals led to higher performance than easy goals, 'do your best' goals, or no goals at all. Provided that the client has sufficient ability to work towards the goal, then a number of factors appear to facilitate goal-attainment. These are: the provision of feedback to show progress towards the goal; support and encouragement from key people such as the nurse; rewards such as money being given for progress; and the acceptance of goals by the individual.

These findings represent a useful set of guidelines for the nurse. Although 'money' seems irrelevant, it is actually not uncommon in hospitals to have formal or informal incentive schemes which give money (or something else that is valued by the client) in exchange for work towards a goal. The *token economy* is a clear example, where tokens (such as plastic discs) are earned by long-stay residents in exchange for the completion of tasks such as self-care routines (shaving, dressing, washing and so on). Nurses have played the main role in operating the token economy, negotiating and reviewing goals or dispensing the appropriate number of tokens (see Higson, (1987) for example).

This example reminds us that goal-setting is also important in helping a unit or service to function optimally. In an ideal world, the place in which help is provided has goals which are closely related to the goals of nurse and client and the whole system is geared up to undertake a common task. Unfortunately much therapeutic endeavour takes place in services and units without this kind of co-ordinated effort. The result can be demoralising for nurses and clients, as goals achieved in therapy are soon lost in the organisational system. For instance, a long-stay resident who is being helped on a one-to-one basis towards a number of goals, all concerned with increasing the resident's autonomy, but who lives in a ward where everything is always done for them, is unlikely to make much lasting progress. But if this individual work were related to a comprehensive ward approach, such as the token economy, then it could be enhanced in effectiveness.

In my own experience, such unit-level goal-setting is both necessary and helpful to all concerned. Over a number of years I have worked in psychiatric day hospitals and, in conjunction with doing one-to-one therapy, have attempted to facilitate a comprehensive, co-ordinated approach. Sometimes the goal-setting is straightforward, as when all the staff examined the reasons why our clients were attending and compared this to what we provided in the unit. This made us realise that we had to develop new programmes. Anxiety was the second most frequent problem referred, yet while we had all sorts of other programmes we had nothing specifically tailored for those clients with anxiety. When the goal-setting is not so obvious, I have found the *Ward Atmosphere Scale* most useful. This brief questionnaire is completed by all staff and clients, leading to a profile of scores representing where the unit or service is at present, and where the staff and clients would like it to be in the future. An illustrative *Ward Atmosphere Scale* is to be found in Chapter 2, while a full account of this kind of systems-level goal-setting appears in Milne (1988). This systems-level analysis highlights another guideline for goal-setters: select as goals those things which are likely to be supported within the client's environment.

Specific goals

Although most nurses and unit managers welcome the idea of goal-setting, relatively few have gone on to clarify what these goals might be. Most of them simply list some of the guidelines for goal-setting, such as clearly stating a small list of realistic goals. To return to the work of Barrowclough and Fleming (1986), they encourage the nurse to consider the client's strengths and needs. 'Strengths' are the things that the client can do, such as 'can walk one mile', while 'needs' are those positively-phrased things that the client should learn to do, as opposed to those things they should stop doing. As far as possible, these strengths are exploited to address the needs.

While this is a useful and individually-centred approach, it leaves unanswered the question of what to select as needs or goals. As was pointed out when discussing needs assessment (Chapter 3), there is no obvious answer to this question. I therefore find it helpful to have an outline of the possible goals in a general sense, before working on goals with an individual client. An example, also discussed earlier (Chapter 4) is the *Clifton Assessment Procedure for the Elderly* (*CAPE*, Pattie 1981), which defines the key goals in relation to the kind of care a client needs. Thus, those clients who are severely disorientated and who are not ambulant or continent are in need of more care than those who are simply disorientated. Knowing the significance of these general categories of behaviour helps me to focus on the most relevant goals with the clients. Similarly, Maslow's (1970) hierarchy of needs has often been promoted in nursing as a general way of thinking about goals. Maslow's hierarchy indicates that physiological needs (food, shelter, and so on) are the most basic, while such needs as those for 'self-actualisation' or personal fulfilment are top of the hierarchy.

A more detailed classification of goals has been generated by Bloom and colleagues (see Bloom, 1956; Krathwohl *et al.*, 1964). Although related to education rather than therapy, these classificatory systems repay attention as models in the clear articulation of goals. They also apply fairly directly to the educational element in some forms of

Table 5.1. *A summary of Bloom's taxonomy of educational objectives within the domain of 'thinking' and as applied to psychotherapy goals*

Goal	Clinical examples
1. Knowledge	Having information about the nature of panic attacks; being able to use the correct terms or to provide facts about a panic attack; knowing what to do about a panic attack etc.
2. Comprehension	Client knows what is being said and can make use of the information, but without seeing its full implications or relating it to other material (interpreting or extrapolating).
3. Application	Being able to see how a general rule applies in a specific situation, as in a depressed client with knowledge of the importance of irrational beliefs realising, while having such beliefs, how they will affect his or her mood.
4. Analysis	When, for example, a client can break down what happened to them in terms of key elements, recognising the relationships involved as in a client making sense of parental behaviour and its effect on his or her behaviour.
5. Synthesis	A client can explain an incident to the therapist in a more coherent or enlightening way than before; or being able to develop a part of his or her own therapy programme from existing elements.
6. Evaluation	Here the client is able to judge the worth of something, as in comparing how well he or she is doing this week as opposed to last week; or in recognising how much tokens are worth in the token economy, or money in the community.

psychotherapy. Bloom's group attempted to articulate goals for each element in the triple response system, namely thoughts, feelings and behaviour. Unfortunately they found the task so gruelling that they only completed the first two. Part of the explanation was that instead of simply classifying goals they tried to arrange them in ascending order, that is, to provide a *taxonomy*. *Table 5.1* gives a summary of their taxonomy of goals within the thinking domain.

Bloom's taxonomy of objectives in the affective ('feeling') domain covered, in ascending order: 'attending' to something (listening); 'responding' to it (pleasure or interest); 'valuing' it (preferring one thing over another); 'organizing' values (that is, seeing how things relate); and having a 'value complex' (a general and integrated set of beliefs).

In practice, Bloom's taxonomy can aid the nurse in defining and selecting goals of an educational kind (for example, what a long-stay client might need to know about money or public transport). It can also help us to think about goals as steps on the way to some general outcome. The most common clinical example of this is perhaps the

Table 5.2 *An anxiety 'hierarchy', being a series of goals to be achieved by the client during therapy. This example is based on a real case of 'agoraphobia'*

Goal:	To be able to catch a bus or train and go around town alone
Step 9	To catch a train to town with a friend and to go into 1 or 2 'easy' (quiet) shops
Step 8	To catch a bus and travel to town and back with a friend, but not go into any shops
Step 7	To catch a bus for a stop or two, with a friend
Step 6	To walk to the shops and enter the easiest one (newsagent when empty)
Step 5	To walk with the dog to the shops (5 minutes) but not to go into the shops
Step 4	To walk for 10 minutes alone and away from the shops
Step 3	To walk for 5 minutes without the dog and away from the shops
Step 2	To walk the dog for 10 minutes, still away from the shops
Step 1	To leave the house and walk the dog for 5 minutes, in the opposite direction from the shops

anxiety hierarchy, being a list of feared objectives or activities arranged in order of difficulty. Just as with an educational objective, the aim is to start with a challenging but manageable goal before moving on to the next one. Therapy (in this case anxiety management) consists of helping the client up the hierarchy towards an improved and adequate level of coping. *Table 5.2* illustrates a typical anxiety hierarchy.

Exercise 5.2: Setting training goals
You might find it helpful to apply some of Bloom's objectives to your own learning as a nurse. See if you can set out some appropriate goals (cognitive, affective and behavioural) in relation to your own training (for example, the application of what you learn as a student to your work as a nurse). Try to also bear in mind the guidelines on goal-setting, such as how you could set up challenging goals.

A case study

This case study is based on a nurse's work with a depressed client in the acute sector of a psychiatric hospital. The client was a 40-year-old man who had been admitted following a period in the intensive care unit of the neighbouring general hospital, having taken an overdose. He was diagnosed by the psychiatrist as having depression. The acute ward onto which he had been admitted defined his difficulties in terms of psychological, physical and social factors. Psychologically the client was regarded as having very little insight into his condition, and of having low self-esteem and a considerable sense of guilt. Physically he was restless (hand-wringing a great deal of the time) with sleep disturbance. Socially, he had some regular visitors and was generally skilled in relating to others. However, his irrational belief that other people had problems as a result of him meant that he had some ambivalence about socialising.

The nurse's analysis of the problem attributed his depression to a history of high and unpredictable stress, in relation to the client's employment as a car salesman. A few years ago the client had been divorced from his wife, and, at around the same time, his two daughters had left home to start work. It seems that these life events came at a time of exceptionally high work stress. His capacity to cope with this stress was therefore undermined by the loss of his immediate family. In place of them he began to abuse alcohol as a way of coping, but this was only partly successful. Latterly he had attempted suicide on several occasions.

From this analysis of the problem, three initial goals were set, one in each of the three assessment domains. Physically, the aim was to reduce the risk of self-harm. This was the most important goal, since all the other goals depended on his continued well-being. Secondly, the nurse intended to increase the client's trust and confidence in the staff (a 'social' domain goal). What was sought was more contact with the staff, preferably initiated by the client, and particularly with the key worker. Another indication that this goal was being achieved would be fewer complaints about the staff 'observing' the client. Lastly, the psychological goal was to improve the client's insight into his depression. Initially he simply attributed it to 'bad luck', but the nurses felt that it would be more appropriate to move him towards the view that there were some controllable factors which might explain his difficulty, such as stress and personal coping strategies.

In terms of negotiation, the nurses in the acute sector often had to lay down initial goals without discussion, due to the client's condition (lack of insight or poor co-operation). This was the case in this example, although the aim was to move towards negotiated goals as soon as possible. This might take several weeks of effort. Once the client takes more responsibility for goal-setting, then appropriate encouragement and reinforcements are offered for working towards these goals. In this client's case, staff encouraged him towards his goals and praised him for any progress made.

The goals of individual clients are consistent with those for the ward as a whole. For instance, the ward worked towards enabling clients to cope more effectively so that they could be discharged successfully. This depended in part on better insight into their difficulties, and in part on having sufficient trust to co-operate with the community psychiatric nurses.

A final point to be illustrated through this case study is the role played by the problem analysis in helping the nurse to respond sympathetically to the client. Because the nurse perceived the depression in terms of such factors as major life events and inadequate coping, he was able to interpret the client's lack of trust or co-operation in a way that encouraged his sympathy and caring. Also, by assessing in a systematic way the nurse was able to develop a better understanding of the client's problem. The client responded favourably to this effort and improved understanding, so encouraging the nurse to continue in this sympathetic manner.

Summary

In this chapter I have advocated a major role for problem analysis. This consists of the definition and explanation for a problem, and is presented as the bridge between assessment and therapy. It was also suggested that the process of problem analysis serves to increase the individuality of clients and to enhance the therapist's capacity to respond sympathetically to challenging behaviour.

Once a problem has been analysed, the next step is to determine some goals, ideally in negotiation with the client. These direct and motivate our efforts, while providing the essential basis for evaluation. Several guidelines are suggested, including the importance of incentives and realistic goals. The case study illustrates how some of these points apply to a depressed man on an acute ward, and also how some of the guidelines, such as negotiated goals, could not be followed in every case.

Questions for further consideration

1 It was suggested that the way we look at things in assessment and therapy is determined by the conceptual model we use. Can you list some examples, drawn from your own clinical experience?

2 Can you now repeat this step, but this time try to adopt a different conceptual model (for example, from cognitive or behaviour therapy)? Once this is done, notice how the two models yield different impressions of the problem and how it might be tackled.

3 Using a conceptual model and clinical problem of your own choice, try to explain why the problem is either caused or maintained.

4 Are the reasons for the cause and the maintenance of a problem always the same? Under what circumstances might they be different?

5 A number of the functions served by goal-setting were suggested (for example, mobilising effort). Try to provide a detailed example of such a function, either from your own learning or from your knowledge of a client.

6 One function of goal-setting is that it makes it possible for you to evaluate. Draw up two lists of goals, one of which you think would make evaluation straightforward, and a second which is in some way problematic. What distinguishes these two sets of goals?

7 Amongst the goal-setting guidelines it was suggested that small, 'challenging' steps were advisable. How can you tell when a step actually meets this guideline?

8 Determine what the goals are on several wards (or for units or services). What are the strengths and weaknesses of these goal statements? Can you suggest any improvements? What do the staff on those wards think of your analysis and suggestion/s?

References

Barrowclough, C. and Fleming, I. (1986). *Goal Planning with Elderly People: How to make plans to meet an individual's needs.* Manchester: University Press.

Bloom, B. S. (Ed; 1956). *Taxonomy of Educational Objectives. Book 1: Cognitive Domain.* London: Longman.

Ellis, A. (1962). *Reasons and Emotion in Psychotherapy.* New York: Lyle Stuart.

Higson, P. (1987). Evaluating Behavioural Interventions in Psychiatric Hospitals. In Milne, D. (Ed.), *Evaluating Mental Health Practice.* London: Croom Helm.

Hokanson, J. E. (1983). *Introduction to the Therapeutic Process.* London: Addison-Wesley.

Kingston, B. (1987). *Psychological Approaches in Psychiatric Nursing.* London: Croom Helm.

Krathowl, D. R., Bloom, B. S. and Masia, B. B. (1964). *Taxonomy of Educational Objectives. The Classification of Educational Goals: Handbook 2: Affective Domain.* London: Longman.

Lazarus, R. S., Averill, J. R. and Opton, E. M. (1974). The psychology of coping: issues of research and assessment. In G. V. Coehlo, D. A. Hamburg and J. E. Adams (Eds) *Coping and Adaptation.* New York: Basic Books.

Locke, E. A., Shaw, K. N., Saari, L. M. and Latham, G. P. (1981). Goal-setting and task performance: 1969–1980. *Psychological Bulletin, 90,* 125–152.

Marks, I. M. (1986). *Behavioural Psychotherapy.* Bristol: Wright.

Maslow, A. H. (1970). *Motivation and Personality.* New York: Harper and Row.

McKie, R. (1990). Sunbathing reduces the risk of breast cancer. *The Observer,* Feb., 18th, 1990.

Milne, D. L. (1987). *Evaluating Mental Health Practice: Methods and Applications.* London: Routledge.

Milne, D. L. (1988). Organisational behaviour management in a psychiatric day hospital. *Behaviour Psychotherapy, 16,* 177–188.

Pattie, A. H. (1981). A survey version of the Clifton Assessment Procedures for the Elderly (CAPE). *British Journal of Clinical Psychology, 20,* 173–178.

Rachman, S. (1977). The conditioning theory of fear acquisition: a critical examination. *Behaviour Research and Therapy, 15,* 375–387.

Stekel, W. (1923). *Conditions of Nervous Anxiety and their Treatment.* London: Kegan Paul.

West, J. and Spinks, P. (Eds; 1988). *Clinical Psychology in Action.* London: Wright.

Further reading

Williams, J. M. G. (1984). *The Psychological Treatment of Depression: A Guide to the Theory and Practice of Cognitive-Behaviour Therapy.* London: Croom Helm. Mark Williams is one of the UK's leading proponents of cognitive therapy, and this readable book is especially valuable for its emphasis on problem formulation from the perspective of various models.

Hokanson, J. E. (1983). *Introduction to the Therapeutic Process*. London: Addison-Wesley.
This is a rare book in that it considers in detail the steps from problem definition to therapy, providing detailed case studies, including transcripts of therapist–client speech and procedural flow charts. Four kinds of therapy are considered: 'supportive', 'behavioural', 'relationship' and 'insight'.

Carnwath, T. and Miller, D. (1986). *Behavioural Psychotherapy in Primary Care: A Practice Manual*. London: Academic Press.
As with Hokanson's book, this offers helpful flow charts suggesting which steps to take in assessment and therapy. It mainly considers the behavioural model (with a bit on the cognitive model), but does so in relation to some basic principles (such as relaxation methods) and a wide range of clinical problems.

Miller, E. and Morley, S. (1986). *Investigating Abnormal Behaviour*. London: Lawrence Erlbaum.
Miller and Morley take a long hard look at depression in this book, dwelling on such major issues as classification, models, epidemiology, life events and a comparison of 'relationship' and 'action' therapies.

West, J. and Spinks, P. (Eds; 1988). *Clinical Psychology in Action: a Collection of Case Studies*. London: Wright.
This is a positive gem – a well-organised and wide-ranging account provided by 40 UK psychologists. Each brief chapter describes a different kind of 'case', mostly consisting of traditional clinical work, but extending to work in organisations. Of most relevance here, each chapter contains a section on formulation.

6 Planning options

The last chapter, on planning tasks, centred on analysing the client's needs in relation to the assessment information. This leads to the question of which resources are available to meet these needs, and is the focus of this chapter. In this respect, nursing is well resourced. The range of psychotherapeutic options available to mental health nurses is vast and confusing. While there are some stalwarts amongst these options, the list of 'new' therapies grows by the day. In addition, refinements of established approaches are promoted regularly and new fashions come along every few years. All this change and development, against a background of continued professional debate and dissent, helps to explain why many of us are bewildered by the therapeutic options.

I was stuck by the sheer range of possible options when on holiday in Santa Fe, a New Mexican town of artists and therapists. The *Santa Fe Sun*'s advertising pages were full of therapy options. On one page I counted over 60 forms of therapy ranging from the familiar hypno-therapy, yoga, and stress management to a variety of therapies of which I knew nothing. Amongst these were: 'integrative body therapy'; 'past life regression'; 'primal therapy'; 'psychic counselling'; 'rebirthing'; 'rolfing'; 'sound healing' and much more. My bewilderment was eased by picking up a book which stated that these unfamiliar therapies represented the 'fourth force in psychology'; that is, they went beyond the familiar behavioural, psychodynamic and humanistic approaches to include the spiritual, intuitive and transcendent aspects of human beings. My training as a psychologist had systematically excluded such aspects from the 'proper' study of human beings, so it is perhaps not too surprising that I was bewildered!

What are your options?

These novel therapies are fascinating and perhaps effective, but we need to consider here the options that are available to you as a nurse working in settings which will almost certainly be less liberal than that of Santa Fe. Indeed, this raises the questions of what the word 'option' means for us. There will be a number of practical and theoretical limitations on the resources you can use

The work context is one consideration, as the number or type of staff

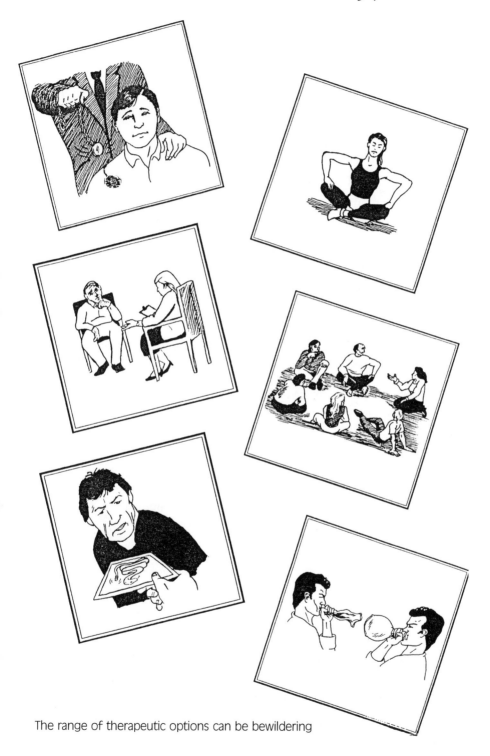

The range of therapeutic options can be bewildering

and clients present will have to be taken into account. In this sense we know that there are insufficient staff to carry out some of the familiar and well-established therapies, such as psychoanalysis; and we know that client groups will respond differently to alternative therapies.

Another consideration is the level of training required to conduct a therapy. For some esoteric therapies, such as the more spiritually-focused ones mentioned above, a personal 'gift' or talent may suffice. Indeed, training in these therapies may be seen as irrelevant or counterproductive. For other therapies there has to be a lengthy period of training, but the majority tend to require one or two years to achieve basic competence, assuming that the trainee therapist has an appropriate educational background and professional qualification prior to any such specialised training. Good examples of such training courses for nurses are those arranged by the English National Board (ENB) or through professional and academic organisations which include 18-month post-registration courses in behaviour therapy.

One consideration when thinking about care plan options, therefore, is the level of proficiency required to implement the plan and the extent to which this proficiency is available in your setting. The multidisciplinary team crops up here, and the skills audit will help you to decide whether other disciplines can be of assistance (for example, by providing a co-therapist). As emphasised in the section on MDTs in Chapter 2, it is important for all concerned to ensure that any therapist is working within the limits of their competence.

Another critical aspect of the therapeutic option appraisal is the extent to which a given approach is of demonstrated value to the kind of client you are dealing with. This raises the question of the theory and research evidence behind the different therapies. As nursing becomes an increasingly research-based profession, there should be a parallel growth in the nurse's concern for the empirical evidence. Alternative techniques should be judged in relation to their proven success, as presented in scientific and professional journals, books and at conferences. Examples of such evidence follow. It will become obvious that the 'fourth force' therapies have neither the theory nor the research base to justify their inclusion in this section, nor, I would suggest, their use by mental health professionals.

A model evaluation

To illustrate the empirical approach to selecting amongst options, a major study on the relative merits of two approaches to psychiatric rehabilitation by Paul and Lentz (1977) compared the value of a psychosocial programme with that of a milieu approach for severely disabled psychiatric clients. The *psychosocial programme* consisted of the application of behavioural methods, such as nurses reinforcing appropriate client behaviour, including the use of tokens. In the *milieu programme* (administered to a matched group of clients in another unit), emphasis was placed on clients making decisions and taking action for themselves, in the spirit of the 'therapeutic community'.

Paul and Lentz continuously assessed staff and clients in both kinds of unit over a period of six years. This included observations of staff–client interactions and evaluations of the client's levels of functioning in a variety of ways. They found very clear evidence favouring the psychosocial programme over the milieu approach (and over the traditional hospital programme) on all important measures, including successful resettlement in the local community and lower treatment costs. They concluded that the psychosocial programme was 'the treatment of choice for the chronically institutionalised mental patient, whether showing severe deficits in functioning, extremes of psychotic and bizarre behaviour, or both' (p423).

Often the kind of clear research evidence that Paul and Lentz (1977) have provided will not be available. Even if it is, there may be good grounds for questioning whether the same results would be obtained in your setting with your client group. This may indicate the need for a local evaluation of the therapy. It would be appropriate for nurses to become involved in such studies, both to better judge the therapeutic options and to foster the research base of nursing. I will resume this theme in Chapters 9 and 10. For the present, please note that such research activity does not necessarily entail special or lengthy training, but rather a curiosity about one's work and a commitment to careful measurement.

Taking the client into account

The last consideration which I wish to emphasise is *client variables*; that is, the ways in which differences between clients (or in the same client over time) can influence the therapy options. In theory we may know that a Santa Fe type list of therapies is available, while recognising that in practice these can have very limited application. For instance, elderly clients with a significant hearing impairment are unlikely to prove good candidates for highly verbal therapies, such as cognitive therapy, even if their major difficulty is identified within the cognitive domain (for example, irrational beliefs). Similarly, such clients may require slower and less strenuous tasks when receiving behaviour therapy such as relaxation training. Woods and Britton (1985) consider several such examples, while also drawing attention to some of the other difficulties that can be encountered when applying therapies to different client groups. Called *treatment socialisation*, these difficulties centre around the client's willingness to accept or participate in a given therapy. The most common example is the widespread preference for medical treatments over the 'softer' psycho-social alternatives, with, for example, anxiolytic medication being preferred to anxiety management. There can therefore be a considerable task facing the nurse who would apply an otherwise suitable therapy. Indeed, to be successful therapy often has to be preceded by an induction or socialisation period, in which the therapist negotiates with a reluctant client. This may be based on sharing information, with the therapist providing details of the proposed therapy and the client disclosing reservations about it.

A case study: An overview of the intervention options

A nurse's help will often be based on the nature of the relationship they have with a client, or on simple alterations to the client's environment, rather than on an intensive form of psychotherapy. A case study will illustrate these often interwoven elements of 'care'. This follows on in many respects from the Paul and Lentz (1977) example, in that the clients were diagnosed in terms of such labels as 'chronic schizophrenia' and the therapeutic option pursued in the ward was akin to the milieu programme. In keeping with this parallel, I will be considering a whole ward as the 'case'.

The ward is housed within the traditional context of a large psychiatric hospital, part of the Mental Health Unit which contains all the case studies in this book. The ward manager also oversees two houses in the hospital grounds, which are part of a 'core and cluster' arrangement. In addition to these basic features of the clients' physical environment, the nurses have given attention to a number of other details. These have included unlocking cupboards and encouraging clients to use the kitchen to prepare their own meals or refreshments. The main aims of the ward are to improve client independence and quality of life, but attempts to do this by re-arranging the furniture in the lounges have proved less successful. However, clients who progress to one of the houses enter an environment that appears to make a very favourable impact on independence and quality of life. There the clients are in a relatively small group of eight, surrounded by all the familiar trappings of a normal home. This is borne out by the clients' families, who are far more likely to visit them when they are in the house.

The favourable effect on clients is illustrated by the case of a 62-year-old man diagnosed as having chronic schizophrenia and presenting with major self-help skills deficits (including such personal hygiene activities as changing underwear and bathing regularly). While he was on the ward there had been no progress, but once in the house he made rapid progress, despite little or no staff effort being directed at these deficits. This points to an influence of the general physical environment on client behaviour.

Another important dimension in helping clients is the therapeutic relationship that is established. In this case, the manager had implemented some of the characteristic elements of the therapeutic milieu. Specifically, he passed over responsibilities at every turn to his clients, encouraging them to problem-solve as a group. Particularly in the house clients were empowered to make decisions and exercise control over all aspects of their own lives, including rules and regulations, shopping and budgeting. After an initial period of the more commonly observed apathy and inertia, he reported that clients moving to the house become far more active and lively, conducting problem-solving conversations amongst themselves about the decisions that they felt had to be made.

The nurse–client relationship in this kind of intervention is therefore akin to that existing between adults, in that each party respects the other's independence and accepts responsibility for their own actions. Role barriers are reduced to a minimum, although the nurses still oversee some 'institutional' routines, such as the provision of two meals a day to the people in the house.

In this sense, the nurse will effectively rely on the quality of the person-to-person relationship, rather than on therapeutic techniques, to promote the clients' quality of life. This is not to say that some distinctive techniques are not blended into the therapeutic milieu (for example, social skills training). But these were all implemented in a low-key fashion, supplementing the milieu approach here and there, rather than representing a major aspect of the overall programme of care.

In summary, this case study indicates how environments, therapeutic techniques and relationships can be combined in a typical setting. Amongst other things it shows how ideas from other programmes are incorporated and adapted as necessary, reflecting the available options.

The option appraisal has included such factors as the needs of the particular group of clients, the physical settings available to facilitate their independence, and the training and therapeutic orientations of the nursing staff. Next I will consider some of these options in more detail, especially how psychology can guide the ways in which an environment can be altered to improve client functioning; and on how individual and group psychotherapies, which emphasise relationships and techniques, can contribute to this process.

Changing the environment

Chapter 2 included a section on how different environmental factors could shape the behaviour of staff and clients. These included physical, social and political dimensions. I went on to consider briefly how the *Ward Atmosphere Scale* could help us to understand and control some of these important environmental factors, for the benefit of all concerned. This present section is intended to elaborate on additional ways in which we can improve the clients' environment, so that these can be considered when planning for their care.

The long-standing but nonetheless profound recognition of the phenomenon of *institutionalisation* is important in highlighting the role of the client's environment. Goffman (1961) is the person most often associated with discussions of what he termed 'total institutions'. In his book *Asylums* he abstracted some of their common features:

> First, all aspects of life are conducted in the same place and under the same single authority. Second, each phase of the member's daily activity is carried on in the immediate company of a large batch of others, all of whom are treated alike and required to do the same things together. Third, all phases of the day's activities are tightly scheduled, with one activity leading at a pre-arranged time into the next, the whole sequence of activities being imposed from above by a system of explicit formal rulings and a body of officials. Finally, the various enforced activities are brought together into a single rational plan purportedly designed to fulfil the official aims of the institution. (p17)

As studies accumulate, it seems that without exception the client's 'disease' is found to interact with their treatment environment, whether we consider the 'physical' or 'mental' conditions of their surroundings. Painfully slowly, it seems to me, those who plan and work in therapeutic environments are putting this knowledge to good use in changing the way in which clients are housed and treated, in order to reduce the features of Goffman's total institution. Although the obvious reference here is to the psychiatric ward, these points are equally relevant to any setting, such as a client's home or sheltered accommodation, as we shall see from the examples which follow.

Making sense of environments

First, consider how we might conceptualise treatment environments. There are many ways of doing this, and again the social-climate scales developed by Moos and his colleagues (for example, the *Ward*

Atmosphere Scale) is a useful model. A more general one, which I think helps us to construe all sorts of environments, has been provided by Pincus (1968) in relation to institutions for elderly people. Pincus distinguished between four dimensions of an environment: public–private; structured–unstructured; resource sparse–resources rich; and integrated–isolated. These dimensions were to be considered in relation to certain aspects of the setting, such as the staffing, physical properties, and procedures. In this way one could consider the extent to which staff accorded privacy to clients (for example, knocking on bedroom doors before entering), or whether a client living in the community was receiving adequate social support.

Changing environments

In discussing the Pincus model, Woods and Britton (1985) provide some examples of research on the effects of altering the therapy environment. One of the key aspects to consider changing is the *social environment*. This refers to staff–client interactions and is probably best considered as the relationship between staff and Pincus' 'structured–unstructured' dimensions. An illustration from Woods and Britton concerns the client's level of 'engagement' in their environment, that is, the degree of client involvement and participation in a setting. They cite studies in which approximately a quarter of clients are 'engaged' at any one time. By altering the nature and amount of activities, nurses were able to significantly increase the amount of client engagement. A good illustration, which shows the interplay between the physical and social environment, is the altering of routines. For example, Quattrochi-Tubin and Jason (1980) considered the effects providing coffee and biscuits in the lounge of a large nursing home had on the participation of elderly people. The aim was to foster a sense of community amongst the residents by encouraging them to participate in gentle exercises and to socialise together. These researchers found that voluntary attendance in the lounge was dramatically increased by this arrangement, as were the social interactions amongst the residents. Further evidence for this effect was a reduction in TV viewing during these exercises and coffee sessions. Some of the elderly people commented that they enjoyed being in the lounge, even though they neither drank the coffee nor joined in the exercises, because they felt part of a group. A subsequent study by Carstensen and Erickson (1986) also showed that simple changes in the therapy environment can dramatically alter client behaviour. They replicated Quattrochi-Tubin and Jason's (1980) study, finding that serving refreshments raised the level of client interaction. But they also addressed the question of whether this increase was a good thing by measuring the quality of client speech during these interactions. They found that the bulk of client speech was 'ineffective' (that is, incoherent or nonsensical), leading Carstenson and Erickson to caution against simplistic measures or interpretations of the effects that follow such environmental changes.

In another example of work with elderly people, Willcocks *et al.* (1987) selected an instrument which emphasised the social environment, including the degree to which clients were able to determine what went on in their institutions and the extent to which they were able to participate in these activities. Four social environment scales were used by these researchers in their survey of residential life in local authority old people's homes. They were:

- *choice/freedom*: the degree to which residents have freedom over their lifestyle (for example, meal times);
- *privacy*: availability of a time and place for oneself or one's friends;
- *involvement*: degree of resident participation in the organisation of home life;
- *engagement/stimulation*: extent to which staff encourage resident autonomy and independence.

Higher scores on these scales indicated a more 'progressive' style of organisation. Willcocks *et al.* (1987) also surveyed ten other variables, including physical amenities and whether the care provided was oriented towards clients or staff. The 100 homes they surveyed varied considerably on their measures. They found, for instance, that small group living, a popular panacea latterly, may yield a better physical environment and provide for more privacy and choice. However, such settings may also have higher levels of worry and lower levels of personal or job satisfaction. They concluded that the variations between homes were considerable, in terms of the physical environment and the organisational style. Despite these differences, Willcocks and his colleagues still noted 'a degree of uniformity which pervades the general atmosphere in all homes' (p138). They also noted that the variations they obtained in the residents 'wellbeing' may have been due in part to their health, personality and past living circumstances, as well as to the institutional setting.

A rather different example concerns the phenomenon of *expressed emotion* (*EE*). This refers to the amount of hostility, dominance and general emotion in the client's environment (for example, the frequency of arguments or critical comments). It has been associated with studies of how those clients labelled as 'schizophrenic' adapt to their return home from hospital. The evidence to date suggests that homes where there was high expressed emotion from the relatives were associated most strongly with clients' relapse and readmission (see, for example, Vaughn and Leff, 1976).

Miller and Morley (1986) provide an interesting summary of research on 'EE', while discussing carefully the concept itself. Amongst their reviewed articles were studies by Leff *et al.* (1982) and Falloon *et al.* (1982) which contained useful ideas for care planning. Both studies were based on systematic work with the families of clients diagnosed as schizophrenic. This included providing them with factual information on causes, symptoms and treatment; developing lower 'EE' ways of coping with daily problems (for example, avoiding distressing clients and providing emotional support); and therapy sessions for the whole family, which were also intended to alter the quality of family interactions. Other interventions have included social skills training and developing problem-solving approaches, both aimed at the whole family. The results from these studies have been promising, with those clients who received the 'EE' package doing better on clinical status and time spent in hospital than control groups.

These examples illustrate the role of people and environments in influencing the client, and they suggest that nurses have a crucial role to play in shaping the client's quality of life. There is clearly scope to develop the ways in which we organise our care. Two points emerge from this brief review of 'changing the environment'. Firstly, nurses will be more or less involved in the various aspects of the therapy environment. Thus, they may not be able to influence the design of a new community home, but by their presence they are inextricably bound up with the quality of care that is provided in settings. This leads to the view that nurses are therapists, at least with a small 't', even if they regard themselves as simply providing 'care'.

The second point which I would like to tease out of this section is that careful evaluation plays a vital part in the development of good therapy environments. While I shall return to this point in Chapter 10, it is worth stressing the importance of the kind of careful scrutiny accorded to a simple environmental change by Carstensen and Erickson (1986). It is this degree of analysis which will provide the basis for the long overdue improvements in environments, and so minimise the features of 'total institutions'.

Individual psychotherapy

The traditions of environmental change and individual psychotherapy have tended to follow two quite distinct paths through the history of clinical psychology. This reflects the rather opposite assumptions each tradition makes about client behaviour, one tending to emphasise the ascendancy of what is *outside* the individual, the other being more interested in the *inside* determinants of behaviour. This rather crude distinction is preserved in individual psychotherapy itself, although there are many shades of grey, as illustrated earlier by the Santa Fe example. Thus, while the behaviour therapists can be seen to be broadly concerned with changing environments, the psychoanalysts can be regarded as focusing on changing people from the inside.

Of course, in reality the differences between the psychotherapies is rarely so clear-cut, with overlaps apparent in both the process and outcome of therapy. This overlap is most striking with regard to outcome, with the many studies of different therapies yielding surprisingly similar results (Stiles *et al.*, 1986). In contrast, studies of the process of psychotherapy suggest considerable diversity, reflecting the different approaches used by therapists. Hardy and Shapiro (1985) have summarised some of the main findings. Client-centred therapists, for instance, tend to use more reflection and acknowledgement in their work; psychoanalysts tend towards more interpretation and questioning; while behaviour therapists tend to use advice and to give information. Such observed differences are consistent with the theoretical bases of these therapies.

Two groups of psychotherapies

Although the psychotherapies can be seen as a collection of quite distinct approaches, there are some common themes which unite large numbers of them. Recognition of these themes can help us to understand therapy process and outcome, thus aiding planning. One theme, apparent in the examples just cited, is concerned with creating a therapeutic relationship within which interpersonal problems can be discussed, including those arising earlier in the client's life. This general approach has been termed *exploratory* psychotherapy. It is identifiable by greater therapist emphasis on interpreting what the client says or does during the therapy session, and on the exploration of what this might mean, in relation to their past. Standing in fairly clear contrast is the *prescriptive* psychotherapy mode. Here the therapist concentrates on what takes place in the client's life outside the session, in relation to their current coping strategies. Little attention is directed at the past, particularly the distant past. In keeping with this emphasis, the therapist would try to enhance the client's coping repertoire, for example training them to relax in the presence of feared stimuli. This therapy mode would encompass cognitive and behaviour therapies, as they share the theme of enhancing such coping skills as relaxation by direct education and training.

Hardy and Shapiro (1985) provided a comparison of these two approaches, observing the work of therapists especially trained in conducting prescriptive and exploratory therapy. A general instrument, the *Helper Behavior Rating Scale* (*HBRS*), was used to analyse what the therapists said to their clients during eight sessions of each form of therapy. They found that therapists in the exploratory mode made significantly more use of interpretation and exploration, whereas during their work in the prescriptive mode they asked more questions and gave more advice and information. Overall, prescriptive therapy was associated with more therapist speech. There were no differences on the remaining six forms of speech measured by the *HBRS*. These findings led Hardy and Shapiro (1985) to conclude that there were indeed large differences between therapies and that these were consistent with the underlying theories, and not simply attributable to personal characteristics of the clients or therapists. Their data also indicate the shades of grey between different forms of therapy, as they failed to find a significant difference between prescriptive and exploratory therapy on the majority of *HBRS* items. For example, there were no obtained differences on such forms of therapist speech as 'reflection', 'process advisement' and 'reassurance'. Definitions of all the *HBRS* items are given in *Table 6.1*, which also includes a summary of the Hardy and Shapiro (1985) results.

Exercise 6.1: Therapy types
As an exercise, you may find it useful to try to code what is said in therapy, using the *HBRS*. It is best to work from a tape or transcript of a therapy session, so that you can consider which therapist utterances belong in which *HBRS* categories. Sometimes tapes or transcripts are readily available locally, or they can be recorded by yourself either in your therapy work or in role-play with a colleague. Hokanson (1983) provides brief therapy transcripts in his book. By analysing at least half an hour's therapy in relation to the *HBRS*, you can work out a rough 'profile' of that therapist. This serves both to clarify the different elements of therapy and to provide detailed information or feedback to the therapist on the type of therapy they were providing. This can be enormously interesting, as I discovered when I applied the *HBRS* to a sample of my own therapy sessions (Milne, 1989). As *Table 6.1* illustrates, my therapy came somewhere in between the prescriptive and exploratory modes.

The 'dodo bird verdict'

In other papers concerned with the *Sheffield Psychotherapy Project*, Shapiro and his colleagues have drawn attention to a major paradox in psychotherapy. This is that despite the clear differences in the therapies provided to clients, they all turn out to be fairly uniformly effective (Stiles *et al.*, 1986). In their own therapy outcome evaluation, Shapiro and Firth (1987) reported that while there were some results favouring prescriptive therapy, in general there were few clear differences in the relative effectiveness of these two forms of therapy. They therefore added evidence in favour of the long-standing 'dodo bird verdict' (Luborsky *et al.*, 1975). This states that 'everybody has won and all

Table 6.1. *Mean percent frequencies of therapist utterances in* Hardy *and Shapiro's (1985) 'exploratory' (E) versus 'prescriptive' (P) analysis and for the present author (DM)*

Response mode	Brief definition	Treatment		
		E	P	DM
Interpretation	Giving client new information about him/herself (e.g. highlighting parallels)	19.6	5.9	8.1
Exploration	Expressing client's previously unverbalized thoughts/feelings (e.g. reformulating)	12.8	3.0	5.9
Reflection	Re-presenting client's message (e.g. paraphrasing)	6.0	5.1	6.1
General advisement	Guiding out-of-session behaviour (e.g. homework)	1.9	12.4	7.7
Process advisement	Guiding within-session behaviour (e.g. suggestions or commands on what clients should do during the appointment)	4.9	3.5	2.4
Reassurance	Responding positively to client (e.g. agreement, praise)	43.8	47.8	40.2
Disagreement	Responding negatively to client (e.g. criticism)	0.6	0.5	0.5
Open question	Gathering unrestricted information (e.g. why do you think you did that?)	1.7	4.4	7.1
Closed question	Gathering specific information (e.g. have you discussed this with your husband?)	2.2	6.9	14.8
Information	New information not about client (e.g. instruction on relaxation)	3.5	7.6	4.2
Self-disclosure	Acts which significantly reveal helper (e.g. recounting a personal experience)	2.6	1.6	1.4
Other	Other types of helper behaviour (e.g. social talk)	0.2	0.9	2.1

must have prizes', following the race verdict of the dodo bird in *Alice's Adventures in Wonderland* (Carroll, 1962).

These various findings indicate that nurses can help clients by adopting general relationship-enhancing forms of speech with their clients. This would include providing lots of reassurance, reflecting back the client's message, and disclosing information about oneself. These forms of speech and the emphasis on the importance of a good therapeutic relationship are common to most forms of psychotherapy. Nurses can also help by adopting more specialised forms of speech, in keeping with their therapeutic orientation and the client's needs. Thus, prescriptive therapists would ask more questions, while exploratory ones would tend to do more interpreting of what the client says or does. Some clients prefer to work in one mode rather than another, so there is a clear indication that planning must take these points into account.

Notwithstanding the 'dodo bird verdict', there are some indications that prescriptive and exploratory therapy do yield different results. Systematic reviews of the clinical outcomes achieved by these therapies suggest that prescriptive approaches may be more effective in the treatment of depression and anxiety, particularly for specific phobias and for obsessional-compulsive disorders (Smith *et al.*, 1980; Stiles *et al.*, 1986). However, outcome research is still in its infancy and it is therefore too soon to claim clear advantages for one kind of therapy over another. Research still has to grapple with the complex interaction of clients, therapists, therapies, problems and settings. This is a major task and will not be progressed significantly in the near future. Nurses who want to design a care plan involving psychotherapy are therefore best advised to carry out their own evaluations, treating the results of outcome research as a guide. In this way they can learn to adapt plans in the light of local experience. Suggestions on how to conduct this kind of evaluation are offered in Chapter 9.

Therapy in written form: bibliotherapy

Nurses are also well advised to consider the written material available for individual psychotherapy. This ranges from general introductions to particular theoretical approaches to highly detailed therapy manuals. Many of these manuals are designed by prescriptive therapists for the client, and can be used independently of the therapist, or in conjunction with therapy sessions. For example, Mathews *et al.* (1981) produced and evaluated two agoraphobia manuals, one for the client and a second for the partner. The manuals were based on a cognitive-behavioural approach, and revolved around *in vivo* desensitisation, pursued in a gradual and systematic fashion.

In general, evaluations of self-help manuals (sometimes called *bibliotherapy*) support their use, indicating that they are reliably more effective than no therapy at all (Scogin *et al.* 1990). I will consider self-help manuals in greater detail in the next chapter, since they offer a simple way of enhancing therapy while minimising any deficiencies in the training that therapists receive.

Group psychotherapy

In a real sense, the earlier discussion of changing therapy environments concerned a literal form of group therapy, as did the case study presented at the outset (p132). However, the term is more commonly used to refer to therapeutic work with small numbers of clients (usually 6–12) in a fixed setting with closed membership, involving the same therapists throughout. As with individual psychotherapy, the therapist's orientation will determine whether the group is basically exploratory or prescriptive. I will again consider both forms of therapy in relation to what is done and how it helps. First I turn to the rationale for seeing clients in groups.

Why have groups?

Discussions of group therapy usually concentrate on the logic behind this approach as far as clients' needs are concerned. To follow Barker (1982), a group affords the client opportunities to share and discuss difficulties with similar others; to obtain support and encouragement; to practise alternative ways of coping; to learn from the coping strategies of others; and to have a structured period of therapist-guided assistance. At the very least, then, it can be seen as providing the basis for social support. Indeed, some of these events seem like ordinary social interactions, but in group therapy they take on new functions. For example, the client can obtain the chance to share in the experiences of others to a degree which rarely arises in social groups. This can be especially important in mental health nursing, as your clients may have developed coping strategies which cut them off from other people (perhaps through social avoidance and the cognitive distortion of events). By gaining a better appreciation of how other people with a common difficulty cope, the group therapy member is also in a position to develop new ways of looking at people and things. A major example lies in their growing capacity to assume the perspectives of others, and so test out beliefs and assumptions about themselves which have been allowed to grow to irrational proportions (for example, 'I'm a freak: no-one else is like me'). Another way in which the psychotherapy group can go beyond an ordinary social group is in providing opportunities for the sharing of genuine reactions to one another. An example here would be the group's acceptance of someone who had always assumed that they would be rejected or devalued by others. These kinds of reasons for groups will of course vary from therapy to therapy, as I will indicate shortly.

Groups can also be organised for purely 'economic' reasons, that is, to provide as many clients as possible with specialised forms of help. As Barker (1982) notes, group therapy can easily conjure up the notion of 'block treatments', in which inadequate resources are fashioned to meet clients' needs under the euphemism of 'group therapy'. That is, there may be an expedient rather than a therapeutic reason for organising groups. In the USA, the group model can also make therapy less expensive and so serve the clients' economic needs too! In a related sense, groups can also serve staff or organisational needs in terms of the training of one or two inexperienced therapists by a group leader or facilitator.

In essence, the reason for organising a therapy group is to create the kind of conditions for learning which other forms of intervention cannot provide as adequately, if at all. Another, economic, reason is to make therapy available to more people than would be possible through individual approaches.

Exploratory group therapies

As with the individual psychotherapies, there are many forms of exploratory group therapy. Well-known examples would include

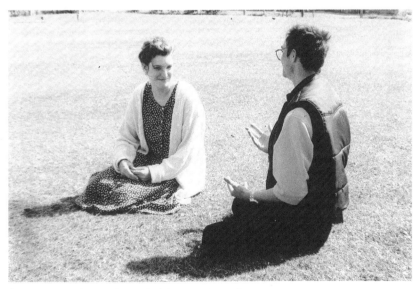

Sharing experiences is central to group work

'sensitivity' or 'T-groups' (also known as 'encounter groups'), and 'psychodrama'. In addition, the main forms of exploratory therapy – psychoanalytic, gestalt, and client-centred – can be conducted in groups. These therapies share as their method the interpersonal relations between the group members. For instance, Moreno, a Viennese psychiatrist credited with coining the term *group psychotherapy* in 1931, had his psychodrama groups act out their feelings as if in a play. In this type of therapy, one client might be asked by the group therapist to play the part of a son and converse with a second client who is asked to play the role of his father. By this means the clients may be helped to express feelings and beliefs which were resistant to individual psychotherapy. Other group members may be involved in staging other dramatic incidents from a client's past, again to help in the process of acknowledging underlying thoughts and feelings. Moreno actually made use of a stage in order to help his clients view life as a kind of drama, taking on the role of 'director' himself to achieve maximum effect.

Because of the nature of these exploratory groups, the general term *interpersonal group therapy* is usually applied. According to Kingston (1987), such groups focus on the 'here and now' experience of relationships amongst group members. They aim to promote personal growth through the interactions which take place in the group, with the result that clients are enabled to enjoy more fulfilling relationships. Kingston highlights four assumptions underlying interpersonal group therapy:

- relationship problems are regarded as central for group members, who either avoid them or encounter difficulties within them;
- clients in groups relate to one another in ways that are similar to their relationships with significant others;
- group members learn from each other how their own ways of relating are seen by others and hear how they affect others;
- the feedback from the rest of the group will help the client to change how they relate to others.

Role of the therapist

The therapist's role is to facilitate these processes by organising the group in the first place and then by helping to create an atmosphere in which clients feel safe to express their feelings about one another or themselves. At different stages the therapist will, for example, summarise and interpret. In sensitivity groups, for instance, the therapists are full group members which means that their own feelings, reactions and effects on others are as legitimate a topic as those of the other group members. However, the therapist may also occupy a distinctive role in commenting on what is going on in the group, or step in to help clients during difficult periods. The therapist will not, though, seek to do this unless it appears necessary, as the observations of the other group members may do most to promote insight. For this reason the group leader will often remain silent (Aronson, 1991). Client-centred therapy groups also use non-directive facilitators. It is assumed that personal growth can occur as clients confront their emotions with honesty, so the therapist's role is basically to clarify feelings. *Table 6.2* summarises some of the main functions fulfilled by group therapists.

Table 6.2 *Basic functions performed by group leaders, following Yalom (1985)*

Function	Definition
1. Emotional Stimulation	Challenging, confronting, active; risk-taking through high self-disclosure.
2. Caring	Offering support, affection, praise, protection, warmth, acceptance, genuineness and concern.
3. Meaning Attribution	Explaining, clarifying, interpreting, providing a cognitive framework for change; translating feelings and experiences into ideas.
4. Executive Function	Setting limits, rules, norms and goals; managing time; pacing, stopping, interceding, suggesting procedures.

Client selection

Participation in group processes obviously places some burdens on the clients, and so some selection of group members is necessary. Kingston (1987) described selecting clients who were likely to benefit from the group, excluding clients who had difficulties making contact with reality or those who were unable to sit peacefully through sessions. Clients were also required to have an interest in participating, and to be likely to contribute ideas to the group; but not to the extent of monopolising it. In addition, the blend of individuals should be considered in such a way as to promote mutual benefits and cohesiveness (for example, by selecting those with similar needs). Cohesiveness is regarded as especially significant, as it gives the group an identity and so helps to promote regular attendance, participation and a willingness to help one another. It usually develops over time, so clients must be in a position to attend regularly for some months. Another selection factor is whether the client is 'psychologically minded', that is interested in developing self-understanding. This will help individual members to arrive collectively at a psychological solution, as opposed to, say, a medical one. These selection criteria are broadly similar for prescriptive group therapy.

Although the therapist may take great care over the selection of group members, certain types of problematic people still appear to emerge in groups. Yalom (1985) identified nine types, including 'the boring patient', 'the help-rejecting complainer' and 'the self-righteous moralist'. To illustrate, the latter has a marked tendency to try and prove they are right and to demonstrate that the other person is wrong. This can generate resentment to the point where the therapist has to provide protection for the client while helping the other group members deal with the provocation of the moralising.

Prescriptive group therapies

These therapies are more likely to stress the importance of acquiring new ways of thinking and behaving in relation to 'there and then' situations. Unlike the 'here and now' focus of interpersonal groups, they are intended to address the difficulties clients face outwith the group, in work or in domestic problems. Group processes are emphasised only in so far as they aid the client's adaptive thinking and behaving, as in modelling one's behaviour on that of the therapist or rehearsing such things as social skills. Thus, the balance in prescriptive group work is on the side of therapy *in* groups, as opposed to therapy *through* the group.

It follows that prescriptive group therapies are less varied in nature than exploratory ones, in the sense that the approaches derive from the principal cognitive and behavioural methods used with individuals. The major exceptions include social skills training and token economies, both of which exploit the group situation in order to promote the clients' learning.

Social skills training

Social skills groups are probably the best known example of a prescriptive model. They are intended to develop the client's capacity to relate effectively to others, helping him or her to become more assertive or to initiate and maintain conversations. Such difficulties are considered to be central to other problems, such as anxiety and depression, and relatively amenable to brief group therapy sessions.

Clients are helped to develop their social skills by means of a systematic programme of learning experiences, controlled by the therapist. The programme might include an initial definition of a specific skill by the therapist, followed by a chance for group members to comment on the degree of difficulty they experience in this skill in relation to real situations they face (for example, expressing opinions). Next, the group might watch two therapists role-playing a way of dealing with this situation, before practising it in pairs themselves. At this stage, the therapist would be providing feedback and encouragement, often with the help of video-tape recordings. In this way clients and therapists can pinpoint and replay difficult situations in order to raise understandings of the finer points of social behaviour, such as eye-contact, posture and gestures.

The therapist's role

It is clear that the prescriptive group therapist takes far more control over the group than his or her exploratory counterpart. As the label suggests, they see it as appropriate to prescribe methods to clients, to the extent of asking clients to complete 'homework' assignments or study carefully prepared hand-outs. This educational emphasis is in keeping with the aim of enabling the clients to learn to understand and behave more appropriately. The assumption is that faulty learning, rather than illness or inadequate insight, is the reason for any observed difficulty.

Evaluation of group therapies

Trying to judge the effectiveness of a group can be more difficult than evaluating individual therapy, since there is the extra 'interpersonal' dimension. This can mean that a group is regarded as successful when its members change their attitudes or relationships to one another in a way that makes them feel better about each other at that time. This may bear no relationship to their thoughts, feelings or behaviours in another time or place. Indeed, the evaluation may be seriously distorted by the very processes that seem to make group therapy work, such as group pressure to conform (in this case to an accepted appreciation of the therapy). In addition, the goals of group therapy are diverse and sometimes unspecified, further complicating evaluation. For instance, in T-groups the aim is to experience things in and about oneself afresh or for the first time. The process is therefore the outcome. In social skills groups, far more specific and objective goals would be identified, lending them to more careful evaluation.

In the early days of exploratory group therapies, there were some reports of promising results, with the clients becoming more interpersonally sensitive, communicative, relaxed and considerate (Aronson, 1991). There were also reports of casualties from T-groups, that is, clients leaving a group having experienced intense yet unresolved feelings. One of the largest evaluations of an exploratory group was conducted by Yalom and colleagues (Yalom, 1985) in the 1970s with students at Stanford University. Expert therapists from ten different forms of exploratory psychotherapy were compared. The results indicated that approximately one-third of the participants had undergone moderate or considerable positive change, in contrast to much less change experienced in a control group. These beneficial changes were maintained for at least six months. However, eight per cent of participants suffered 'psychological injury' lasting the same period, and they were part of the two-thirds majority who did not benefit. Yalom and colleagues concluded that the range of encounter groups which they studied were not a highly potent agent of change.

Yalom's team was also able to shed light on the effectiveness of different leadership styles, the main focus of their research project. They found clear and positive relationships between 'caring', 'meaning attribution' and positive outcome: the more these therapist qualities were present, the better the results. In contrast, 'emotional stimulation' and 'executive function' had a curvilinear relationship to outcome: too much or too little of these leader behaviours resulted in lower client outcomes (see *Table 6.2*). To illustrate, a therapist who exerted too little of the 'executive function' – a laissez-faire style of leadership – resulted in a bewildered, floundering group; too much 'executive function' produced a highly structured, authoritarian group, which therefore failed to develop either autonomy amongst its members or a freely flowing interactional style. A case of Plato's 'golden mean' again being true, at least for 'executive function' and 'emotional stimulation'. The most successful therapists moderated these two functions, while offering high levels of 'caring' (offering support, acceptance, and so on) and 'meaning attribution' (explaining, clarifying, interpreting).

Prescriptive group therapies have been more amenable to evaluation. The first major text on social skills training (Trower *et al.*, 1978) contained a review of outcome studies in which both in- and outpatients were regarded as benefiting, as measured by a range of instruments. The out-patients appeared to benefit most, indicated by more lasting improvements in such areas as an extended social life and an accompanying reduction in their need for therapy. Trower and his colleagues concluded that there was evidence from controlled studies that social skills training improved skills, that these were lasting and were relevant to real life situations. In addition to confirming these conclusions, Ellis and Whittington (1981) noted some advantages of social skills training over comparable interventions. These included: the generally positive experiences of clients; the relative brevity and low cost of training; its proven usefulness to a wide range of clients; and high rate of acceptability to clients.

Summary

I have provided an account of the planning options available in mental health nursing in terms of three interrelated levels of activity: the therapeutic environment, the individual and the group. In turn, the case study illustrated how these can overlap with client variables to yield some complex challenges to the nurse as care-planner. In considering the three levels, I elaborated on the message presented earlier that the environment in which clients live plays a major part in their wellbeing. Important dimensions include the degree of privacy, structure and involvement which are present in a setting. These can sometimes be manipulated by nurses, often with remarkable results.

Individual and group psychotherapy take place in environments characterised by these dimensions, but they are usually set apart to a noticeable extent, having special rooms or staff. Both forms of therapy are extremely variable and defy the kind of brief overview that is possible in a book of this kind. I have attempted to deal with them by emphasising the distinction between prescriptive and exploratory psychotherapies, while noting a shared base in the blend of a therapeutic relationship with distinctive therapy techniques. Despite often dramatic differences in these techniques, and the theories underlying them, there is a paradoxical equivalence in their respective effectiveness.

Group psychotherapy extends work with individuals by affording clients special opportunities to develop their skills in relationship enhancement. Group facilitators appear to use the same broad types of behaviour as in individual work, with somewhat comparable results. Group work is therefore worth considering when planning care, not least because it can be an efficient use of scarce resources and a productive way to engage clients in self-help.

Questions for further consideration

1 What determines the range of realistic care plan options available to a mental health nurse? Discuss with reference to one setting in which you have worked.
2 'Treatment socialisation' refers to the extent to which a client is prepared to collaborate with therapy. How might this be increased?
3 Nurses often emphasise a 'caring' as opposed to a 'therapeutic' role, but can these be separated?

4 In this chapter, the very broad distinction has been drawn between 'prescriptive' and 'exploratory' psychotherapies. List as many different individual therapies as you can think of, then see if you can find another way of grouping them.

5 How might you explain the 'therapeutic paradox' (that is, that apparently diverse therapies produce seemingly equivalent outcomes)? How could your explanation be tested out?

6 Yalom (1985) has suggested a number of different 'types' of group therapy member (for example, 'the self-righteous moralist'). What would you regard as the strengths and weaknesses of classifying clients in this way?

7 Supposing you were running an 'exploratory' form of group therapy, how might you set about evaluating it?

References

Aronson, E. (1991). *The Social Animal,* 6th edn. New York: Freeman.

Barker, P. J. (1982). *Behaviour Therapy Nursing.* London: Croom Helm.

Carroll, L. (1962). *Alice's Adventures in Wonderland.* Harmondsworth: Penguin Books.

Carstensen, L. L. and Erickson, R. J. (1986). Enhancing the social environments of elderly nursing home residents: are high rates of interaction enough? *Journal of Applied Behaviour Analysis, 19,* 349–355.

Ellis, R. and Whittington, D. (1981). *A Guide to Social Skill Training.* London: Croom Helm.

Falloon, I., Boyd, J., McGill, C. W., Razin, J., Moss, H. B. and Gilderman, A. M. (1982). Family management in the prevention of exacerbations of schizophrenia: a controlled study. *New England Journal of Medicine, 306,* 1437–1440.

Goffman, E. (1961). *Asylums.* Harmondsworth: Pelican.

Hardy, G. E. and Shapiro, D. A. (1985). Therapist response modes in prescriptive vs exploratory psychotherapy. *British Journal of Clinical Psychology, 24,* 235–245.

Hokanson, J. E. (1983). *Introduction to the Therapeutic Process.* London: Addison-Wesley.

Kingston, B. (1987). *Psychological Approaches in Psychiatric Nursing.* London: Croom Helm.

Leff, J., Kuipers, L., Berkowitz, R., Eberlein-Vries, R. and Sturgeon, D. (1982). A controlled trial of social intervention in the families of schizophrenic patients. *British Journal of Psychiatry, 141,* 121–134.

Luborsky, L., Singer, B., and Luborsky, L. (1975). Comparable studies of psychotherapies: Is it true that 'everyone has won and all must have prizes'? *Archives of General Psychiatry, 32,* 995–1008.

Mathews, A., Gelder, M. G. and Johnston, D. W. (1981). *Agoraphobia: Nature and Treatment.* London: Tavistock.

Miller, E. and Morley, S. (1986). *Investigating Abnormal Behaviour.* London: Lawrence Erlbaum.

Milne, D. L. (1989). Multidimensional Evaluation of Therapist Behaviour. *Behavioural Psychotherapy, 17,* 253–266.

Paul, G. L. and Lentz, R. J. (1977). *Psychosocial Treatment of Chronic Mental Patients: Milieu versus Social Learning Programme.* Cambridge, Massachusetts: Harvard University Press.

Pincus, A. (1968). The definition and measurement of the institutional environment in homes for the aged. *Gerontologist, 8,* 207–210.

Quattrochi-Tubin, S. and Jason, L. A. (1980). Enhancing social interactions and activity among the elderly through stimulus control. *Journal of Applied Behaviour Analysis, 13,* 159–163.

Scogin, F., Bynum, J., Stephens, G. and Calhoon, S. (1990). Efficacy of self-administered treatment programmes: meta-analytic review. *Professional Psychology: Research and Practice, 21,* 42–47.

Shapiro, D. A. and Firth, J. (1987). Prescriptive v Exploratory psychotherapy: outcomes of the Sheffield Psychotherapy Project. *British Journal of Psychiatry, 151,* 790–799.

Smith, M. L., Glass, G. U. and Muller, T. I. (1980). *The Benefits of Psychotherapy.* Baltimore: Johns Hopkins University Press.

Stiles, W. B., Shapiro, D. A. and Elliott, R. K. (1986). Are all psychotherapies equivalent? *American Psychologist, 41,* 165–180.

Trower, P., Bryant, B. and Argyle, M. (1978). *Social Skills and Mental Health.* London: Methuen.

Vaughn, C. E. and Leff, J. P. (1976). The influence of family and social factors on the course of psychiatric illness. *British Journal of Psychiatry, 129,* 125–137.

Willcocks, D., Peace, S. and Kellaher, L. (1987). *Private Lives in Public Places.* London: Tavistock.

Woods, R. T. and Britton, P. G. (1985). *Clinical Psychology with the Elderly.* London: Routledge.

Yalom, I. D. (1985). *The Theory and Practice of Group Psychotherapy,* 3rd edn. New York: Basic Books.

Further reading

Bloch, S., (Ed; 1986). *An Introduction to the Psychotherapies.* Oxford: University Press.
Eleven eminent therapists provide accounts of a range of approaches, including brief focal psychotherapy, crisis intervention and family therapy.

Dryden, W. (Ed; 1990). *Individual Therapy: A Handbook.* Milton Keynes: Open University.
Fifteen authors describe their different therapeutic approaches, ranging from the familiar (such as person-centred) to the rare (such as Kleinian, Jungian and Adlerian therapy). Each chapter covers the history and development of the therapy in the UK, followed by a statement of the model and the main techniques that are employed.

Kuipers, L. and Bebbington, P. (1987). *Living with Mental Illness.* London: Souvenir Press.
This is a book intended to help relatives and friends to cope with someone with mental illness, specifically schizophrenia and manic-depression. It provides information, explanation and useful tips on coping.

Reynolds, W. and Cormack, D. (Eds; 1990). *Psychiatric and Mental Health Nursing.* New York: Chapman and Hall.
Another collection describing different therapies and also a range of nursing models. Contributors first discuss the theory, then provide examples of clinical applications.

Warr, P. (1987). *Work, Unemployment and Mental Health.* Oxford: Clarendon Press.

This scholarly review considers how the environment, including one's employment status, influences wellbeing. Many of the environmental features found to be important can be seen in individual and group psychotherapies, not just in the general environment (for example, interpersonal contact and control). Warr also provides an analysis of the interaction between individuals and environments.

Wilkinson, J. and Canter, S. (1982). *Social Skills Training Manual*. Chichester: Wiley.
This helpful book is written for those who would like to introduce social skills training with their clients. Assessment, programme design and running the training programme are covered in considerable detail.

SECTION FOUR

Implementation

7 Direct work

In the preceding two chapters I addressed some of the tasks and options facing the nurse in preparing a care plan. These chapters were fundamentally theoretical in character, in the sense that they detailed all manner of possibilities and considerations. In this (and the next) chapter I intend to move on to consider the *action* or *implementation* phase of the nursing process and shift our focus towards some of the practical aspects which determine the level of care that is actually provided. As will become evident, however, theory and practice have much to offer one another, so we will often have reason to refer back to the 'planning' chapters in particular.

Theory and practice

How should we think about the implementation of care plans? What model might guide us to raise useful questions, or help us to see possible answers? Stockwell (1985), in her discussion of care plan implementation, drew attention to a number of potentially important factors. These included the nurse's freedom to conduct the plan in a flexible manner, the availability of supportive colleagues and the opportunity to do interesting work. Barker (1982) highlighted the available resources, the need to assign clear responsibilities and the training needs of the nursing staff. Dexter and Wash (1986) emphasised the need for identification of the client's goals and sensitivity to both client and environment.

Although these all seem like eminently sensible considerations, the differences between the authors illustrate the lack of a widely accepted or comprehensive model for considering care plan implementation. If nursing is to fulfil the promise of Project 2000, at least in the sense of becoming a research-based profession, then models should be drawn from the empirical literature rather than from personal experience, as these authors appear to have done. Such a research-based model should help us to construe the task of implementation and suggest some fruitful approaches. The way of thinking is guided by theory, thus reflecting a scientific approach; the approaches we consider and apply are practical, yet they can also test out theory.

A model of implementation

I will now try and illustrate this mutually enriching cycle between theory and practice by adopting a suitable model for this chapter – this is Warr's (1987) model of work, based on his review of relevant literature in sociology and psychology, which indicates the role of nine features of a job in determining how well it is performed. These are listed in *Table 7.1*, together with some definitions intended to show their relevance to mental health nursing. As these are general features of work, they should, if the theory is sound, apply to nursing. The case study, based on these job features, is a way of testing out the model. All the implementation issues which Stockwell (1985), Barker (1982) and Dexter and Wash (1986) identified are present, and the additional headings which I had intended to address, such as client compliance with therapy are readily assimilated to Warr's model. So the model fulfils the requirement that it should help to explain and integrate different things, while deriving from a research base. This base also guided me to raise particular questions, and afforded some possible answers from the previous studies of work on which it was founded, as well as directing my attention to particular research within nursing.

In this chapter I will therefore consider each of Warr's work features in relation to the job of implementing a care plan. As before, a typical case study provided by a nurse will be used to discuss these features. This time the case is the work of a nurse with a ward of elderly people, and I will relate this to each of the headings which follow.

The opportunity for control

This is regarded as probably the single most important feature of a job, in the sense that most of the job's remaining features are to some extent dependent upon it. Three aspects of control are distinguished in *Table 7.1*: decision-making, motivation and predicting the consequences of decision and action.

Making decisions

Much of what was covered in the last two chapters is relevant here (decision-making is also discussed in the foundation text to this series: Niven, 1993). Nurses need to weigh up possible options against real practicalities, and make a decision concerning the kind of care to provide. The nursing process aids decision-making by emphasising the role of successive care plans guided by regular evaluation. Thus, any one decision has to be viewed in the light of this series, or process, of decision-making.

Table 7.1 *A list of the main features of a work environment, after Warr (1987)*

Work environment features	Definitions related to psychiatric nursing
1. Opportunity for control	The ability to control activities and events, as in making decisions, being motivated, and being in a position to predict the consequences of a care plan.
2. Opportunity for skill use	Nursing skills can vary in terms of the extent to which they are used or developed. They are important for goal attainment and job satisfaction.
3. Externally generated goals	Work can consist largely of imposed demands and requirements for routine duties. These can limit the range of care plan goals that are possible.
4. Variety	As the number of novel roles available to nurses increases, so repetitiveness and other negative features of jobs decrease.
5. Environmental clarity	Good working environments have some predictability, clear role requirements, and have some form of feedback on the extent to which nurses do a good job.
6. Availability of resources	The demands of implementing care plans need to be balanced against the available resources, including staffing ratios, staffing range, and adequate physical options (for example, a group therapy room).
7. Physical security ('Health and Safety')	Work is promoted when nurses have a secure place to carry out their duties (and which is safe, warm and so on).
8. Opportunity for social contact	Nurses need to share their work with one another and with other staff members in order to obtain social support, motivation, co-operation and the opportunity to compare practices.
9. Valued social position	A nurse's work should be capable of earning respect from others as a result of its importance, status, calibre.

In order to make good decisions about care, nurses have to be in a position where they can exercise some control, since the decisions usually imply the use of some resources. This control might concern access to rooms or equipment; the predictability of their shiftwork;

their influence over other staff, such as specialist therapists; or their ability to gain the client's collaboration. Key words related to control from Warr (1987) are *autonomy, discretion, power* and *influence*. He emphasised that typically these will vary with different aspects of one's work, and that members of large organisations, such as nurses, are unlikely to have complete control, making decision-making problematic. This implies that decisions should take into account the nurse's degree of control over a care plan. In some respects this control may be fairly complete, as in *intrinsic control*, where decisions only affect one's own immediate work. Altering details of a client's care plan which you are administering as key worker would be an example of high intrinsic control. However, in implementing the plan you might find that the client is exercising some kind of *counter-control*. That is, they are trying to exercise control over you! A study of this process showed that patients were able to effect a significant degree of control over the decisions nurses were able to make (Sanson-Fisher and Jenkins, 1978).

In contrast, decisions requiring greater *extrinsic control* (that is, influence over other people's work or resources) would be more difficult to make or regulate. These points bring to mind the literature on innovation in organisations, as this similarly concerns attempts to control people and their environments, usually at the level of altering policies and procedures. Research has tended to indicate the importance of two factors, namely the *content* and the *process* of an innovation (see, for example, Fairweather *et al.*, 1974). In terms of content, it seems that successful changes are based on simple, effective and sustainable changes. In contrast, sophisticated 'high technology' approaches to problems tend to be avoided or abandoned. An example might be a complicated model of nursing. Similarly, the process by which any such change is introduced will tend to make a big difference to its success. Key elements include the involvement of a small group willing and able to support the innovation. The group members do not necessarily need to have high status, and student nurses can play a significant part.

Innovation guidelines can help nurses to increase their control over change, thus enabling them to effect their care plans. For instance, in a psychiatric rehabilitation ward the ward manager evolved his own 'low technology' version of the nursing process. This was successfully implemented, apparently because it met the sort of innovation criteria listed above (Milne and Turton, 1986). This included a clear and straightforward approach to the nursing process, based on the nurses' views about the main priorities. This approach allowed the nurses to control both their work and the demands made on them by managers and others.

Motivation

Feeling that you are in position to decide about the nursing care you provide will have a beneficial effect on your motivation, as illustrated by the preceding example. I have also discussed how a sympathetic model of care can help nurses to work energetically with difficult clients (see Chapter 3). Again, the client's contribution is critical, as he or she needs to believe that your care plan is going to benefit them. Motivation also derives from a sense of achieving success, as when the goals of a care plan are attained. Again, this will tie in with decision-making in the selection of challenging goals which will make reaching them seem like an achievement to the client.

Motivation also increases when our environment reinforces us for the work we do. This can take many forms, for example, in the positive reactions of significant people to our care plans. Managers and peers, for example, often turn up amongst the list of things determining how much work is done, or how well it is executed. In another study of innovation in psychiatric rehabilitation, Burdett and Milne (1985) interviewed nurses in order to ascertain which factors they regarded as important in motivating their involvement in the changes. The support of their manager, relevant in-service training and the client's response to the new therapy were perceived as the most important motives, while insufficient feedback, rules and regulations and lack of equipment were regarded as the main things undermining their motivation. The nurses were able to influence most of these factors by, for example, informing managers of the care plans they were undertaking (including placing charts on the office walls) and of their success. This can free resources and elicit support and feedback from managers.

Nurses' motivation has also been researched in relation to a wide variety of factors, including such incentives as extra time off work, feedback of results, peer support, self-monitoring and prompts such as phone call reminders and posters. Some of these factors were necessarily under the nurses' control while others were the responsibility of the researchers or managers. A clear implication from this research is that individual nurses can play a significant part in controlling their work environment.

Predicting consequences

Control and prediction are the hallmarks of science, in that a 'good' experiment predicts the link between a carefully arranged situation and a certain outcome. In nursing practice it is, of course, rarely possible to establish the laboratory scientist's degree of prediction, given our limited control over many 'real-life' variables. However, we still engage in judgements about whether a certain programme of care will lead to a certain consequence. To the extent that such predictions can be made accurately, we increase our sense of control.

The main consequence to consider is the impact of a care plan on a client. Our knowledge of the efficacy of a given care plan would influence our prediction of the outcome, and so we would want to be familiar with the evidence supporting that particular intervention. For example, in the last chapter we noted that social skills training is effective, as a rule, with out-patients, but less so with in-patients. We would also wish to consider any results obtained from prior care-plans with the same client, and to take account of any other relevant information.

Broadly speaking, four kinds of impact are logically possible, assuming that there is some kind of positive consequence of a care plan. These are the extent to which changes in the client extend across time, people, settings and behaviour. These consequences are referred to as *generalisation*. To illustrate from the social skills training literature, a five-year follow up of the members of a social skills group revealed that improvements had been maintained over this period, a very important consequence of the therapy. Similarly, some group members felt better able to relate to others in home and work settings, and were able to control their anxiety as well as their social behaviour (West and Spinks, 1988). These consequences relate to the four types of generalisation just mentioned.

Unfortunately, mental health researchers do not usually go to this degree of trouble in considering therapy outcomes, but they need not be difficult to judge in relation to many clients and care plans. If they can be considered, they greatly enhance our understanding of the impact of the care we provide, helping with prediction and our sense of being in control of our work.

To turn to the case study, working with elderly people introduces special biases into the issues of 'control'. For nurses working with those with a dementia, motivation may prove problematic because of the client's limited capacity to respond favourably to care plans. However, the ward manager I talked to believed that the nurses had considerable opportunities for control. Their key worker system provided the basis for the implementation of care plans. When a client is admitted, one nurse, the key worker, takes prime responsibility for carrying out a total assessment. This comprehensive appraisal provides the basis for discussion amongst all the ward's nurses on the strengths and needs of each client. This leads to decision-making about the nature of the initial care plan. Client's plans are reviewed regularly, again involving the key worker and the rest of the nursing staff in decision-making.

In addition to exercising control over the individual care plans, the nurses also have the power to determine activities for groups of clients. For instance, they introduced a beauty therapy session for some clients, with the aim of involving them more in taking care of their appearance (for example, using make-up; hairstyling).

In terms of staff motivation, the blend of a key worker system and participative decision-making led to high levels of involvement and commitment. Additionally, staff motivation was facilitated further by refresher courses on various topics and by the successes nurses achieved with their care plans. Predicting the consequences of these plans had become fairly straightforward. There was an emphasis on simple and achievable goals, with only modest expectations of the clients in order to keep ambitions in check.

Exercise 7.1: Implementing a care plan
Using the headings and examples of *Table 7.1*, work in a small group in order to consider the implementation of a specific care plan. This might be one from a ward you all know well, or it could be based on a group interview with an experienced nurse. Each person should select 1 or 2 work features and in turn:

● try to establish how these work features influenced the care plan, and
● try to generate some practical ways of improving the implementation of the care plan.

The case study material presented under each work feature provides an example of how your information might look and a comparison point for discussion in your group.

Opportunity for skill use

Warr's (1987) work environment features are basically all 'desirable', in the sense that they tend to be present to some degree when good work is being done. However, he points out that they can be present to such a large extent that they undermine work performance. 'Skill use' is a clear case in point. Nurses who have no opportunity to use their skills will suffer, but so will the work of nurses who exceed their competence. Those who have the chance to exercise and develop their skills will have the highest job satisfaction, and those who have the appropriate skills will be more successful in attaining work goals.

The largest piece of research which I have undertaken with nurses involved an examination of the effect of an in-service training course in behaviour therapy on the work of rehabilitation nurses (Milne, 1986). As such, it looked at developing the nurses' skills in conducting care plans and the related impact on a wide range of outcomes, including goal attainment and job satisfaction. The course lasted for five days and covered those aspects of behaviour therapy which were relevant to the work of the nurses who attended it (for example, how to design and implement a behavioural care plan). I obtained convincing evidence that the course had significantly improved their knowledge, attitudes and skills, and that this had generalised over a period of at least one year. Turning to the issue of goal-attainment, evaluation of the work of these nurses indicated that this development of their skills was associated with better care planning and implementation. For example, the trained group of nurses were able to write and conduct better care plans than they had been able to prior to the course, and their clients also benefited more from these care plans following this training, as there were better results and more care plans were implemented.

On the issue of job satisfaction, nurses were interviewed following the course and reported that it had made their work more interesting (82 per cent of nurses affirmed this), led to greater feelings of competence (64 per cent) and improved their work skills (79 per cent). Informally, the nurse managers said that the course had helped to raise staff morale, while a questionnaire survey and absenteeism–sickness data bore out the impression of higher job satisfaction.

The provision of further training can therefore enable the use and development of nursing skills. As stressed elsewhere in this book, so can good use of the nursing process (in the sense that the evaluation can serve as feedback to the care planner), co-therapy work, and other options. The real issue, it would seem, is the extent to which a work environment encourages the use or development of skills. Again, this is partly under the control of the nurse (see the preceding section) and partly inherent in the work system. The challenge in care plan implementation is to balance these in such a way as to achieve the goals and so derive satisfaction from the effort. In this sense, all nurses can participate in decisions about skill use and skill development. Students are in a particularly interesting position, as they can often help to keep others abreast of new developments.

In our case study ward, the high level of nursing control meant that staff could use all their skills. Developments in these skills took place in a variety of ways. Qualified nurses always worked in tandem with their unqualified colleagues, in order to pass on skills and ideas. The qualified nurses learnt from attendance at in-service workshops, in an informal but valued way from the student nurses who passed through the ward, and from discussions with other nurses on other wards. The ward manager felt that they had little opportunity to learn from professionals from other disciplines, as they had little presence on the ward.

Externally generated goals

Warr (1987) indicated the significance of goals by drawing attention to the way in which they give rise to plans, which then structure how we behave. As we start to pursue work goals, we tend to test our environment by seeking feedback on our progress towards goal attainment. Goals and plans are therefore seen as a product of the individual nurse and the work environment. An environment that makes no demands on a nurse sets up no objectives and provides no extrinsic motivations, whereas a setting that makes challenging goals can have the opposite effect. Clearly there are dangers in both extremes, as excessively difficult, vague, numerous or imposed goals can destroy planning and motivation (see Niven and Robinson (1993) for a discussion of such problems as 'burnout' and 'alienation'). Such goals are usually referred to as *demands, obligations* or *requirements*.

Research reviewed by Warr indicates that low or very high work demands generally have adverse effects, while goals generated by workers promote attainment and motivation, provided that they are realistic and fit within the overall job and environment. This raises the spectre of conflict between staff as a result of opposing pressures to select or pursue certain goals. Once again, the innovation literature offers some relevant guidelines. Items to consider are:

- *Outside intervention*: usually some 'outsider' with an active, personal and frequent involvement helps to ease conflicting pressures by acting as a facilitator and catalyst (for example, the psychologist attending ward meetings).

- *Participation*: a mix of people (across disciplines, status and so on) involved in participative decision making can help to balance the environmental demands against your care plan goals (for example, the multidisciplinary team can help you to prioritise a ward's work: other nurses can help a student make time to set appropriate goals or can provide useful feedback).

- *Active diffusion*: if you are able to demonstrate useful goal attainment with clients, this can serve to influence managers and others to make different demands in future (for example, it can persuade them to give you more time for your successful work with clients).

The guidelines also suggest that your goals are more likely to be acceptable if they involve an inexpensive, flexible and compatible form of intervention: that is, one consistent with existing values and resources.

The case study has already illustrated the importance of careful goal-setting by the nurses in controlling their own work and in promoting their motivation. Interestingly, the ward manager provided a spontaneous example of the value of outside intervention when she recounted asking a psychologist to help her to address the negative attitude nurses held towards their clients when she took over the ward. This 'outsider' had helped her to argue the need for individualised care plans, giving her an ally and an external reference point.

However, the ward had been subjected to a succession of externally generated goals. These included the nursing process, nursing models and, at the time of our interview, nursing standards. Although often desirable developments in themselves, these innovations were definitely imposed on the ward, sometimes with little negotiation, flexibility, training or support. This inevitably created some bad feeling and resistance on the part of the staff, who saw it as 'just more paperwork'. In addition, these innovations came along at the rate of about two a year! Other external influences had been much more favourable, such as the reduction of client beds to 20 (plus three holiday relief ones) as a consequence of a re-organisation of the hospital.

Variety

Research studies suggest with great consistency that a certain amount of variety in one's work helps productivity, motivation and job satisfaction (Warr, 1987). It is probably a good thing, therefore, to exercise your full repertoire of work skills, in order to achieve these outcomes. In the absence of variety, workers usually introduce 'distractors', such as practical jokes and conversation, which help to pass time but which further reduce productivity.

In these respects, mental health nursing has come a long way in a short time. From being the 'handmaidens' of psychiatrists and the occupants of a relatively low position in the organisational 'pecking order', nurses have risen to positions of autonomy and power, as indicated by this chapter's case study. While this seems to vary considerably from setting to setting, the existence of ward managers with clinical nurse specialists and budgets represents a fairly dramatic increase in the status of nurses. This sets the scene for greater job variety and all that goes with it. In addition to these developments, nurses have undertaken increasingly specialised training for roles which would have been unthinkable a decade ago. I refer to the various advanced courses available to nurses, leading to the kind of varied, independent practice traditionally associated with psychiatrists and psychologists. The nurse therapist is a case in point (see, for example, Marks, 1985).

There is, therefore, considerable and unprecedented variety in the nurse's role, including aspects of 'manager' and specialised 'therapist'.

Occupancy of such roles can help in the implementation of care plans and the variety of work that is undertaken. But for the less rarified roles, there may well be less freedom to undertake different kinds of tasks and less opportunity to exercise a variety of skills. For some people this is not problematic, as they prefer a predictable, routine job. For others, and I assume this represents most students and junior members of the profession, there is a need to find ways to influence job variety. Presumably this arises from many of the other job features (such as levels of control and skill) as well as emerging from the diverse nature of the role (refer to Chapter 2 for a list of seven roles within the nurse's role).

In practice, as the case study has shown, nurses can exercise their control and skills to optimise variety in their work. In her four years in post, the ward manager in this case study has herself changed the nature of her work considerably, particularly in developing the way the ward runs so as to incorporate new ideas and successful practices. For instance, the qualified staff have designed a teaching package which they use with students and nursing assistants, and the total assessment mentioned earlier has come from trying out different assessment instruments and incorporating the best ones into a package. Not least, the care plans are all individualised, which, together with the emphasis on close relationship between nurses and clients, leads inevitably to some job variety.

Environmental clarity

Care plan implementation can be expected to vary in keeping with the predictability, role requirements and feedback of a work setting. By 'predictability' I mean how well nurses understand what will happen and what is required of them. In relation to the above points on the relatively rapid developments of the nurse's role, the predictability of the job can be low. As a result of rapid and continuing change, some nurses may experience a tension between the wish for variety and the need for predictability. One should note that these job features are not incompatible, in that it is possible to have a predictable caseload in terms of number and type of clients, but to exercise a range of skills with the clients one sees. It is also possible to thrive on an unpredictable role, particularly where this fits in with new clinical developments or emerging philosophies (such as 'embracing change') and where this is supported by your peers and managers. The optimal balance may be best approximated by regular discussion with managers and multidisciplinary team members, as they will be in similar positions to you and may be able to increase the predictability of your work. This could well be true for both what is happening, and what is required of you, in your role.

Another dimension of environmental clarity is the extent to which you receive feedback on your implementation efforts. Partly this should come from the evaluation phase of the nursing process with each client, and partly it may come from colleagues (for example, the MDT during case discussions). Both of these can help you to judge your work for yourself. However, a work environment should also provide you with information on your efforts. Recall that nurses in the study summarised in 'the Opportunity for Control' section of this chapter regarded the lack of feedback on the work they and their colleagues were doing as a disincentive to implement their behavioural care plans. The same conclusion emerges from Warr's (1987) review, where he stated that: 'Feedback about action outcomes is a minimum requirement for the establishment and maintenance of personal control and for the development and utilization of skills' (p146). In this respect we look to service managers to set up ways of letting staff know what is required of them and how well they are doing (implementing, perhaps, regular review meetings and annual appraisals). Staff can also collaborate with managers on the provision of feedback by working on such things as 'quality assurance' projects or by joining 'quality circles' to discuss ongoing work. Indeed, one quality assurance project is to set up ways of feeding back information to yourself and to colleagues by means of simple, prompt and clear indications of work performance, such as choosing daily goals in implementing care plans and monitoring your own performance in achieving them (see, for example, Greene *et al.*, 1978; and Burgio *et al.*, 1983). These points are every bit as true of students as they are of more senior nurses.

On the case study ward, the handover discussions about clients and care plans were complemented by regular ward meetings at which information was exchanged, and policy matters or other business was discussed. These served to promote environmental clarity in such areas as role clarification. Feedback on work was, however, less direct, as praise and other forms of appreciation were rare. Nurses preferred to judge their work standards from more natural forms of feedback, such as the continued accreditation of the ward by the nurse education centre, what students working on the ward said about relative standards of care around the hospital (and what the staff themselves knew of this), together with the success they regularly experienced in implementing care plans.

Availability of resources

Warr (1987) focused on money when he analysed this job feature, but it also seems to apply strongly when translated into the more general category of 'resources'. In the present context, these would include people (staffing ratios and expertise) and things (rooms and equipment). I will focus on people.

Considering the availability of people as a resource, the obvious group that comes to mind are other nurses, followed by other professionals. In this sense, we require some help if we are to make a good job of care plan implementation. We need time and space, and we also need guidance and encouragement. Systems such as 'key worker' or 'primary nursing' are understandable in this light. Not only do they carve up the staffing resources so as to meet the demands of client care, but they also afford nurses the opportunity to develop a therapeutic relationship and to follow through with care plans. These points are clearly important in terms of some of the earlier features we discussed, such as environmental clarity.

In addition to one's nursing colleagues, there are the resources of other professionals to consider. As I outlined in Chapter 2, teamworking can at times represent more of a demand than a resource, but team members do have the potential to offer a different perspective, to collaborate on care plan implementation (as in co-therapy with a group of clients), and to apply their skills directly. This kind of collaboration opens up the sometimes considerable resources of other disciplines. However, it can also open up various professional 'sores', such as the 'skillmix' question of the appropriate level of involvement for different disciplines with different skills and proficiency levels. Many psychologists, for instance, have major reservations concerning what they regard as the use of psychological methods by non-psychologists. Some of them feel that only psychologists have the requisite background and training to carry out anxiety management or social skills training, for instance. To take an extreme example, Lewis (1984) has suggested that 'giving psychology away' leads to a dilution or abuse of the methods of clinical psychology, due to insufficient training and supervision. Nurses have their own 'sores', as will be mentioned. Such issues are prominent in these times of rapid role expansion and the erosion of traditional working arrangements.

The sensible answer to such resource difficulties is as far as possible to resolve them by thorough discussion and, ideally, by observation of what others actually do: how often do we clear up misunderstandings of this kind when we gain a full grasp of what the other person means? One person's 'anxiety management' can be another's 'social skills training'. Even when there is overlap, surely there is enough work to go round! If not, this is an opportunity for someone to increase their job variety, either by developing higher levels of proficiency at the given skill or by branching out into other skills (see Niven, 1993).

The client as a resource

I mentioned earlier that other staff were the obvious resource. We should not forget the potential of our clients as self-helpers, and the role of the nurse in fostering this resource. Many care plans will be designed towards this end, so what problems need to be considered here? The earlier phases of the nursing process are highly relevant, in that challenging, negotiated goals and a sound problem analysis will promote self-help. The main issue that comes to mind is that of *compliance*, defined as the extent to which a client's behaviour coincides with the nurse's prescription.

Much research has been conducted on client compliance, including the contributions made by forgetting and misunderstanding. For example, studies of medication use indicate that even among those clients who appear to remember and understand something, between 25 per cent and 66 per cent take the wrong dose and up to 30 per cent make potentially dangerous errors (Niven, 1989). Important factors to consider are:

- complexity of the therapy procedure
- degree of change required in the client's life-style
- length of time for which the advice has to be followed
- whether the condition is very painful
- whether the therapy is seen as potentially life saving
- perceived severity of the problem.

However, many other factors can play an important part, such as the quality of the client–therapist relationship and the role played by the client's family or friends. Niven (1989) summarises the guidelines emerging from research. The ones which seem most relevant to mental health nurses include giving simple instructions and checking that they are understood (sometimes writing them down to help); clarifying the client's expectations and concerns; and, above all, being friendly, sensitive and understanding.

Returning to the case study, we have already seen that the ward for elderly people makes relatively little use of non-nurses, and that it has had a significant reduction in beds. Staffing ratios are adequate and predictable. It was in terms of the physical resources that the ward manager expressed the greatest concerns. She had been promised some furniture to help in the design of a quiet reminiscence room but this had not yet materialised. The decor of the ward was subject to external control, and so she could not influence the choice of wallpaper or carpeting. Although nominally the budget holder, some of the ward manager's minor expenditures were queried by her line manager. These kinds of resource difficulties contrasted with the ward's normal approach of participative decision-making and internal control.

Physical security

This job feature refers to such concerns as protection against physical threat afforded in one's work, and the provision of a comfortable environment in which temperature, noise, fumes, lighting and so on are controlled. Its more common label is 'Health and Safety at Work'. Deficiencies in these areas can impair performance of one's duties, cause discomfort and fatigue, or lead to physical injury, such as back problems from continuous or incorrect heavy lifting.

In comparison with the environments referred to by Warr (1987) (textile mills with high humidity and temperatures, and lint-saturated air), it would seem that nurses have relatively comfortable working lives. However, because of the many windows in the case study ward, exposure to the sun and wind can cause considerable variations in the ward temperature. These are not always accommodated by the hospital computer controlling the central heating, and so it can be uncomfortably hot on occasion.

A second example, which can make mental health nursing more exacting than the textile mill, concerns violence against staff by the client. The ward manager said that she and her colleagues were often 'thumped' by the old ladies in their care, and clients could also be violent to one another. However, she pointed out that such actions were usually followed by a kiss or a hug in the next moment.

Dealing with aggression

Dexter and Wash (1986) provide a useful summary of the various forms of aggression which nurses may experience (including verbal abuse and self-mutilation) and offer some practical suggestions on minimising such difficulties. Amongst their suggestions for dealing with violence is the improvement of the client's coping strategies, thus enabling them to deal more appropriately with strong negative feelings. This could be done by teaching better communication skills or by giving more time to communication or relationship building. If necessary, restraint is used to control an incident.

Breakwell (1989) has emphasised the importance of *predicting* aggression as a way of dealing with it. From a review of the literature, she generated a 'dangerousness checklist' for practitioners to use prior to entering a risky situation.

Amongst the factors likely to increase aggression were the client's status (for example highly stressed, drunk, or with unrealistic expectations), the client's past behaviour (past violence predicts future violence), and the client's situation (are there others present who will encourage or support aggression?). Once you are face-to-face with a client there are some additional predictors of aggression. Breakwell lists:

- the client showing signs of atypical excitement or passivity;
- presence of weapons or similar cues to violence in the room;
- a breakdown in the normal pattern of nonverbal communication (body language, lack of eye contact);
- the client showing signs of rapid mood swings;
- the client being oversensitive to suggestions or criticisms.

She suggests that certain circumstances will increase the risk of aggression. These include working alone with no way of raising the alarm, being in a situation where you can be trapped if the client becomes violent, and being unaware of the cultural norms which regulate the client's behaviour.

In terms of handling a potentially violent outburst, Breakwell recommends that you try and give the impression of being calm, controlled and confident, as far as possible continuing to talk in a normal tone of voice. Instances where the aggressor is attempting to establish dominance can be controlled by feigning submission or by diverting attention (offer to make a cup of tea, for example). If the aggression is inevitable, check on your escape routes or your sources of assistance and try to increase the availability of these options. Breakwell gives the example of overcoming the tendency of bystanders not to help by making a specific request for assistance to a specific bystander. Of course, in the ward situation there should be more readily available assistance, but it is still useful to have an agreed system for signalling alarm and dealing with it. In secure environments such systems would include personal alarms, room alarms and videos monitoring isolated areas. Owens and Ashcroft (1985) have written a helpful book in relation to reducing violence which offers detailed accounts of biological, social and psychological perspectives on the causes of violence.

Opportunity for social contact

I have already considered several illustrations of the way in which nurses can share and compare work practices in order to aid their sense of co-operative working. Warr (1987) cites some classic studies showing how these kinds of interactions tend to improve morale and motivation. He suggests that two kinds of interaction can be distinguished, namely those that are *task centred* and those that are *social-emotional*. In the first of these, nurses co-operate to solve problems by comparing experiences, offering advice, or providing practical help to one another. They may also afford one another social-emotional contact by exchanging information about family, finances or personal difficulties. Nursing may also provide friendships and opportunities to socialise outside of work. These represent the social support functions discussed in Chapter 2, which were seen as a complement to personal coping strategies. While that section was concerned with clients, the coping model also applies to staff. Of particular relevance is the role of social support in providing nurses with a buffer against the emotional demands made by clients. All too often staff are expected to listen to other people's problems without any recognition of their own needs. Offloading these 'hassles' of work with a sympathetic colleague can make the work more tolerable. Another example is the need to express feelings of fear or anger after dealing with an aggressive or violent incident. This appears to be a very common way for people to cope, and is more effective than bottling it all up or avoiding work stressors. Although there can be a tendency to view social support seeking as a form of professional weakness, strong acknowledgement of its importance comes from senior nurses (for example, Altschul, 1983) and from research on 'burnout'. This suggests that supportive communication with colleagues is vital in enabling staff to produce good quality work (McIntee and Firth, 1984).

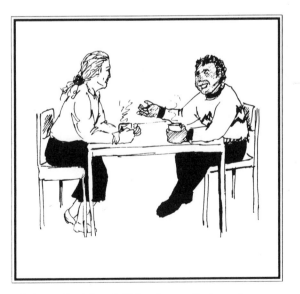

It is important for staff to discuss their work

Valued social position

The final feature of work concerns the esteem it earns from others, as a reflection of its importance, status or calibre. Warr (1987) points out that society largely accords esteem on the basis of one's job, and that this can have an indirect impact on the worker's mental health, for better or worse. For example, social support can vary depending on what you do for a living, as some of Warr's (1987) illustrations indicate (for example, bank clerks and receptionists tend to be ignored at parties!). He points out that esteem can also emerge from colleagues' evaluations of the job or from one's own personal valuations (including those of the service one provides). In these senses, nursing may be seen as capable of earning considerable esteem because it is interesting and provides a valued social service (caring for people with an 'illness').

In the ward manager's opinion, qualified nurses have come to value their position more highly in the last few years. She instanced their greater self-sufficiency, their enhanced skills and their larger therapeutic role. Against this there were some external controls which limited their position, as in the earlier examples of requirements to implement regular changes. She believed that other professionals had mixed perceptions of the nurse's status. Occupational therapists and physiotherapists seemed to resent role overlaps in such areas as responsibility for taking particular groups or taking the clients for exercise, and this seemed to reflect their view of nursing as a less valued position. Others, such as the psychiatrist, accorded them more status and respect.

Relatives of clients seemed to be the most enthusiastic in recognising the nurse's role, partly because they themselves had often had to try and cope with the clients before handing over to the nurse. This helped them to appreciate the nurse's skills, especially in improving the client's level of functioning (for example, reinstating speech or mobility). The clients seemed to hold the staff in high regard too. The ward manager believed that her clients showed their appreciation by cuddles or hand squeezes when unable to express their esteem verbally.

Overall, the ward manager thought that nurses enjoyed the support of the general public, who were impressed by their dedication. She believed that they regarded nursing as a profession and gave it due status, unlike some of the other health service professionals!

Summary

The aim of this chapter was to take a thorough look at the implementation of care plans. This was in order to gain an impression of the important factors determining what work is done, and to review some ideas on more effective implementation. Warr's (1987) book on work provided a likely model for this exercise. Its nine job features were considered in relation to care plan implementation, and these features help to indicate the major determinants of nursing work, while simultaneously illustrating how models derived from research can be applied to nursing practice, an objective of Project 2000.

In terms of facilitating the implementation of care plans, a number of promising options were considered, some derived from a case study of a ward for elderly people. These include ideas from the literature on innovation as a way of securing necessary resources (for example, adopting low technology methods and pursuing them in a participative way), and suggestions for fostering clear and prompt feedback on work efforts. By taking a thorough look at the task of implementing care plans, and by considering these kinds of options, nurses can help themselves to help their clients.

Questions for further consideration

1 Organisational change is a complex phenomenon. From your experience, or from discussions with senior nurses, what are the important determinants of an innovation in psychiatric nursing (for example, the 'nursing process' or 'nursing standards')?

2 How do nurses receive feedback on their work? Can you suggest some practical ways to improve the quality and the quantity of this feedback?

3 Why do you think that clients fail to comply with instructions? What do you see as the implications of non-compliance?

4 How can a student nurse gain more control over his or her work? Try to give practical examples based on the points made earlier in this chapter.

5 To what extent are you given the opportunity to use your skills when you work on a ward? How would you know when you were exceeding your competence?

6 I have argued that the real issue in implementing care plans is not more training but a better work environment. Can you list some examples where this seems to be true and some others where it does not? What would you conclude from these examples?

References

Altschul, A. (1983). The consumer's voice: nursing implications. *Journal of Advanced Nursing, 8,* 175–183.

Barker, P. J. (1982). *Behaviour Therapy Nursing.* London: Croom Helm.

Breakwell, G. M. (1989). *Facing Physical Violence.* Leicester: BPS Books (The British Psychological Society) and London: Routledge.

Burdett, C. and Milne, D. L. (1985). 'Setting events' as determinants of staff behaviour: an exploratory study. *Behavioural Psychotherapy, 13,* 300–308.

Burgio, L. D., Whitman, T. L. and Reid, D. H. (1983). A participative management approach for improving direct care staff performance in one institutional setting. *Journal of Applied Behaviour Analysis, 16,* 37–54.

Dexter, G. and Wash, M. (1986). *Psychiatric Nursing Skills: A Patient-Centred Approach.* London: Croom Helm.

Fairweather, G. W., Sanders, D. H., Tornatsky, L. G. and Harris, R. N. (1974). *Creating Change in Mental Health Organisations.* Oxford: Pergamon Press.

Greene, B. F., Willis, B. S., Levy, R. and Bailey, J. S. (1978). Measuring client gains from staff-implemented programmes. *Journal of Applied Behaviour Analysis, 11,* 395–412.

Lewis, P. (1984). The teaching of clinical psychological skills to non-psychologists. *Newsletter of the Division of Clinical Psychology,* (British Psychological Society) *45,* 32–35.

Marks, I. M. (1985). *Psychiatric Nurse Therapists in Primary Care.* London: Royal College of Nursing.

Mathews, A. M., Gelder, M. G. and Johnston, D. W. (1981). *Programmed Practice for Agoraphobia: Client's Manual.* London: Tavistock Publications.

McIntee, J. and Firth, H. (1984). How to beat the burnout. *Health and Social Services Journal, 94,* 166–168.

Milne, D. L. (1986). *Training Behaviour Therapists: Methods, Evaluation and Implementation with Parents, Nurses and Teachers.* London: Croom Helm.

Milne, D. L. and Turton, N. (1986). Making the nursing process work in mental health. *Senior Nurse, 5,* 33–34.

Niven, N. (1989). *Health Psychology: An Introduction for Nurses and other Health Care Professionals.* Edinburgh: Churchill Livingstone.

Niven, N. and Robinson, J. (1993). *The Psychology of Nursing Care: A foundation text.* Leicester: BPS Books and London: Macmillan.

Owens, R. G. and Ashcroft, J. B. (1985). *Violence: A Guide for the Caring Professions.* London: Croom Helm.

Sanson-Fisher, R. and Jenkins, H. J. (1978). Interaction patterns between inmates and staff in a maximum security institution for delinquents. *Behaviour Therapy, 9,* 703–716.

Scogin, F., Bynum, J., Stephens, G. and Calhoon, S. (1990). Efficacy of self-administered treatment programmes: meta-analytic review. *Professional Psychology: Research and Practice, 21,* 42–47.

Shapiro, D. A. and Firth, J. (1987). Prescriptive v. Exploratory Psychotherapy: Outcomes of the Sheffield Psychotherapy Project. *British Journal of Psychiatry, 151,* 790–799.

Stockwell, F. (1985). *The Nursing Process in Psychiatric Nursing.* London: Croom Helm.

Warr, P. (1987). *Work, Unemployment and Mental Health.* Oxford: Clarendon Press.

West, J. and Spinks, P. (Eds; 1988). *Clinical Psychology in Action.* London: Wright.

Further reading

Cormack, D. F. S. (1983). *Psychiatric Nursing Described.* Edinburgh: Churchill-Livingstone.

This is a rare objective account of what psychiatric nurses actually do, in relation to their clients' needs. Cormack highlights 'effective' and 'ineffective' nursing work. Interestingly, a critical incidents technique is used to describe what is done by nurses.

Dexter, G. and Wash, M. (1986). *Psychiatric Nursing Skills: A Patient-Centred Approach*. London: Croom Helm.
The skills and knowledge base of psychiatric nursing are reviewed in relation to fourteen different kinds of presenting problem, including depression, overactivity and aggression. Practical care plan ideas are detailed for each of these problem categories.

Firth, H. and Britton, P. (1989). 'Burnout', absence and turnover amongst British nursing staff. *Journal of Occupational Psychology, 62*, 55–59.
Firth and Britton conducted a long-term analysis of the relationship between such variables as role ambiguity and perceived support from superiors on the factors in the article's title. They concluded that emotional exhaustion and lack of perceived support both influence motivation, whereas ambiguity about the limits of authority leads nurses to avoid situations.

Bowers, L. (1989). The significance of primary nursing. *Journal of Advanced Nursing, 14*, 13–19.
'Primary nursing' has risen in popularity, Bowers argues, as a result of nursing's search for professional status, together with other forces (for example, a system for implementing the nursing process on a ward.)

Stocking, B. (1985). *Initiative and Inertia: Case Studies in the NHS*. London: Nuffield Provincial Hospitals Trust.
Stocking discusses the literature on innovation in the NHS, particularly how it starts and diffuses through the organisation. In addition, there are four detailed case studies, covering innovations in Regional Secure Units and patients' waking times.

Towell, D. and Harries, C. (Eds; 1979). *Innovation in Patient Care*. London: Croom Helm.
In many respects, this complements Stocking's text by providing more detailed accounts of change in such areas of nursing as care of the elderly, leadership, autonomy, management and training. Another appealing feature of this book is that, like the present one, it reflects work undertaken in one Unit (Fulbourn Hospital, Cambridge).

8 Indirect work

A case study

When Mr Jones started attending the day hospital, he had already
spent six months as an in-patient as a result of alcohol abuse. In the
admission interview he described difficulties in coping with relationships at home and at work, manifested in bouts of panic followed by
social avoidance, and also a sexual dysfunction. He had been helped
to control his drinking during his spell as an in-patient and was now
at the day unit two days a week for continued support. The referral
note had not mentioned the difficulties at work, although Mr Jones
had resumed his job as a mechanic on a part-time basis. Moreover,
on further questioning it appeared that the staff on the acute ward
had focused their attention on Mr Jones in isolation from his family
and colleagues: it had been expected that the combination of
medication and group therapy would suffice.

This example is intended to illustrate some of the major issues
which should be addressed in care plan implementation, such as the
communication between staff in different units, the 'social
boundaries' of a problem like alcohol abuse, and the related task of
involving family or others in a care plan. It is likely that a client like
Mr Jones would receive further benefits from nursing care if
something were done to address these issues, for example involving
his wife in sexual and marital therapy.

The overall aim of this chapter is to take a closer look at some of these
issues, as well as at the nurse's role in caring for the client's carers, in
educating relatives, and in supporting those who provide social
support. These examples are all referred to as *indirect work*, which can
be defined as efforts to achieve health care goals by influencing the
care provided by others. The most common form of indirect influence
is through carers and other staff, although other options can be
relevant. These include evaluating services and using the data to
change how people are cared for, health education or training and
teaching, or changing a system or environment. I will now present
some of the arguments for indirect work.

If indirect work is the solution, what is the problem?

Many services are locked into tradition-bound ways of working: psychologists see their out-patients in GP surgeries, while nurses mostly see their clients in NHS settings. Similarly, mental health units have their day hospitals, while multidisciplinary teams are seen as the only possible way of organising the work tasks. This kind of devotion to tradition can blind us to some rather basic questions, and lead to somewhat irrational service provision. In order to see alternatives, it can be helpful to go back and review 'the problems' solved by the above practices. For the psychologist, this might be to focus on the widespread need for coping assistance amongst the general population, rather than construing this in terms of a long waiting list. For the nurse, 'the problem' could consist of insufficient alternatives. If day hospitals are a Unit's way of addressing the need for transitional phases of care, what else would serve?

So, what are the problems which indirect work solves? As our 'Mr Jones' example indicated, these include ineffective communication, underutilisation of social resources, a limited assessment of his problems, and the limited extent of his therapy. In addressing some of these issues, indirect work can also represent a way of implementing community care policies, a strategy for easing staff shortages, or a more efficient way of providing nursing care. Let me now argue in favour of these bold assertions.

There is a better way!

My impression of the community care movement has been that staff of all disciplines support its principles, although doubting its motives; that is, they see it as being concerned with political ideology and financial gain, rather than with client benefit achieved through better resources. There appears to be agreement that it is a 'good thing' to move towards increased self-help or independence in 'normalised' settings; however, the progress of the movement has been hampered by such obstacles as the inadequate retraining of staff in approaches which are relevant to community care. These approaches will tend to differ markedly from those which operate in psychiatric institutions, in such areas as the need to work more through other people in order to help the client; or in having to consider a wide range of non-institutional settings for the work. 'Indirect work' of this kind is a promising way of implementing community care.

There are some additional arguments in favour of an indirect model of care, including:

- *Prevention*: by working with those people, such as parents and partners, who may directly influence the developments of psychological problems, it is sometimes possible to anticipate and intervene at far less cost to all concerned;

- *Effectiveness*: related to the prevention argument is the one which states that it is only by working through natural relationships (for example, work–colleagues; father–son; boss–employee) arising in their normal environments that we can expect to have any real effect. After all, these are the contexts in which problems have emerged, and so anything approximating to a cure necessarily has to take place in this context. If we take someone out of their context (for example, into hospital), any changes may simply be temporary or due to a break from stressful relationships.

- *Impact*: even were we able to cure people by taking them out of the context of their problem, how many would we be able to help? There are vast amounts of unmet mental health need in the community, and specialist therapy alone cannot meet this need. Surveys suggest that there is a great need to help GPs manage such things as sexual–marital, phobic and obsessional–compulsive problems. Two major UK studies found that 14 per cent of all GP consultations indicated 'psychiatric morbidity' (Shepherd *et al.*, 1966), while a figure of 9 per cent was found for a random community sample (Goldberg and Huxley, 1980). *Table 8.1* summarises the kinds of mental health problems identified by GPs. In short, there are huge numbers of people and a wide range of problems to be addressed by mental health services, and traditional approaches are inadequate to meet their needs.

The 'triadic' model

The traditional approach to these problems has been specialist therapy on a one-to-one basis, founded on the doctor–patient or *dyadic* model of care. Given the low ratio of specialists to people with problems, there need to be other ways of organising a service in order to have more impact. The *triadic* model is one such option, in which the specialist tries to provide help through another person, referred to as a *help mediator*. There have been many successful examples of implementation of the triadic model including such mediators as nurses, carers and partners (see Bernstein, 1984). I will be considering some research illustrations later in this chapter, but for the present, *Table 8.2* provides further details of the model.

The table indicates that different roles (such as nurse, wife, nursing assistant) can have different relationships within the triadic model. In

Table 8.1 *A breakdown of the kinds of mental health problems seen by GPs (Robson* et al., *1984)*

Problem category	Percentage of clients with a mental health problem
1. Anxiety/stress (including phobias and obsessional compulsive disorder)	47
2. Interpersonal (including sexual and marital difficulties)	17
3. Habit disorder (including eating disorders and alcohol dependencies)	16
4. Depression	14
5. Educational and occupational	2.5
6. Psychological adjustment to physical illness (including pain)	2.5
7. Neuropsychological	1.0

Table 8.2 *Some examples of the triadic model*

Specialist	Mediator	Client
Nurse Therapist	Mental Health Nurse	Psychiatric Client
Clinical Psychologist	Care Attendants	Elderly People
General Practitioner	Wife	Husband
Community Psychiatric Nurse	Family	Psychiatric Client
Mental Health Nurse	Nursing Assistant	Psychiatric Client

some instances they may be the 'specialist', that is, the person who has some expertise or resources to supervise the care provided by the mediator. At other times, the nurse may be the mediator, particularly on psychiatric wards where they have a long-standing relationship with the client. The mediator is someone who has this kind of special relationship to the client, together with the willingness and capacity to collaborate on a care plan.

Next I will consider some of the main difficulties and methods of indirect work.

The challenge of effective communication

Good communication is essential for successful collaboration, whether amongst nurses in implementing care plans as part of their direct work, or between nurses and their care-plan mediators (see Niven and Robinson, 1993). As such, it might profitably have been discussed earlier in this book. However, indirect work raises special challenges and so this may be the best place to address the issues raised in communication.

By definition, communication is the passage of a message (that is, some kind of information) from a sender to a receiver. The 'passage' can take various forms, principally the spoken and written word, but often includes nonverbal communication such as facial expressions and gestures. Communication can also vary with respect to its function: it may be informing or persuading the receiver. In this sense, teaching and health promotion are different functions of communication. Other purposes served include encouraging, questioning, criticising and reassuring.

Of course, the nurse is more often concerned with communication as a way of sending messages (such as giving nursing orders or advice), and receiving them (as when listening to or empathising with clients). For all professionals there is a long history of concern over this task, reflecting the complexity of this apparently straightforward phenomenon and its vital role in working life. This is exemplified by the noncompliance with medical advice in the last chapter and the case study at the start of this one. Another illustration comes from research on general nurses' recognition of their clients' worries. This suggests that communication is poor, leading the nurses to overestimate the number of worries to a level threefold that identified by the clients themselves. This poor communication is attributed to the clients' reluctance to interrupt the nurses' activities, hence other patients are better able to estimate the worries. The practical significance of the miscommunication includes excessive reassurance from nurses to their clients (Johnston, 1982).

These findings underline that communication is vitally important and therefore merits special attention if you are to implement care plans successfully. This is especially true when working indirectly, due to greater than usual differences between 'senders' and 'receivers', not to mention unusual 'mediums'. Let us now consider these elements with a view to pinpointing some challenges and some good practices.

Sending messages

Tomlinson (1985) provides a detailed breakdown of communication skills in relation to a number of barriers. She identifies such nonverbal skills as touch, facial expression, personal distance and speed of movement; and verbal skills, including the use of clear and precise language, tone of voice, volume and speed of speech. These elements are usually combined in different ways to convey a given message. An example is a client who uses rapid speech and threatening gestures to communicate, thus signalling anger to the nurse.

The written word shares some of these verbal elements (for example, clear nursing orders), but the absence of the nonverbal cues places greater pressure on the sender to communicate effectively. A further difference is that in speech we can easily put things in different ways. Together with other 'padding' technically referred to as the *redundancy element* in language), this makes it easier to communicate when talking. In these respects we would not normally write as we speak, thus increasing the probability of miscommunication.

Other obstacles to sending messages effectively may include the respective backgrounds of sender and receiver, as when nurses and clients are of different ages, races, genders, cultures, and social classes. These factors tend to promote rather different kinds of speech or writing, including their form and content. They may also determine the kind of help provided to clients (Sayal, 1990).

In essence, it appears that the effectiveness of communication decreases as the distance between the respective cultures of the participants increases, a finding that also holds for subcultural differences such as 'generation gaps' (for example, between an adolescent peer group and their parents). The major explanation for this finding is that the respective assumptions and expectations of the participants often differ. In order to clarify these unspoken assumptions it is necessary to understand the culture of the communicator. This is hard to do, as some of the subtleties of communication are never really discussed or even recognised. An example is the distance two people maintain when conversing, which is quite different in Western and Arab cultures. Other culturally-based differences are more striking, as in the conventions in the USA and Brazil regarding appointments; in the USA someone who is never late for an appointment is seen as more successful than someone who is sometimes or always late, whereas the opposite holds in Brazil. People from these two cultures will therefore tend to differ in their behaviour and in how they interpret that behaviour, both forming a poor (and erroneous) impression of the other. The implication when dealing with people (even those from a slightly different subculture) is to clarify important assumptions and interpretations about one another's behaviour, and as far as possible to develop an understanding of the other's culture or subculture. (Bochner, 1983)

Sending messages also involves some decision about the content and form of a message. The content is the first decision to make. The difficulties of informing relatives about a setback in a client's condition illustrate how taxing it can be deciding what to say. Again, individual differences in such areas as social class and age may shape the nature of the message. Furthermore, in nursing deciding what to communicate may be a group activity. Group decisions bring into play factors which may significantly alter the content of a message. These include the biases introduced by conformity to group norms and compliance with strong leaders. Sometimes groups may also polarise views, emerging with noticeably more risky or more cautious decisions than would be expected from the respective individuals. Niven (1989) describes these processes and provides some interesting exercises to illustrate them.

The form of a communication can differ depending on the physical sense at which it is directed: speech is directed at hearing and writing at sight. It can also differ in the way the information is presented. To illustrate, in trying to promote compliance one might utilise *persuasive communication* techniques such as ingratiation (that is, increasing how much you are liked prior to a compliance request), guilt induction, or obedience to authority. Other form features include the strength, duration and frequency of a message.

Receiving messages

Communicating something to someone else involves many of the elements just mentioned as sending and receiving are interdependent in many respects. This is indicated by such verbal factors as clarity and speed of speech, and by nonverbal ones like eye-contact and speed of movement. In addition, obstacles emerge from an interaction between two or more people with respect to colour, class and so forth (again, see Sayal (1990) for a discussion of these issues). There are also features of the receiver which operate independently. As the senses are involved, then any impairment, such as deafness or partial sightedness, can obstruct good signals.

Obstacles to effective communication

Tomlinson's (1985) useful review also includes a list of variables which can reduce the effectiveness of communication, and which can operate at the individual or group level. These are divided into:

- *psychological variables*, including attitudes, trust, defensiveness, resentment, anxiety and prejudice;

- *organisational variables*, such as roles, rules, regulations, tasks and opportunities; and

- *physical variables*, of the kind recently mentioned (that is, deafness, blindness, noise, smell).

These lists are not exhaustive, making clear the complexity and challenge of effective communication. How can this challenge be met?

Guidelines for effective communication

The preceding outline of 'sender' and 'receiver' variables indicates a number of suggestions for improving communication. Amongst these are matching sender and receiver characteristics to ensure communication to the appropriate sense in the appropriate way (for example, by speech to a sight impaired carer). Other general guidelines include the use of clear brief messages when writing, but longer ones when speaking, to allow for repetition. However, the most important guideline of all is an empirical one: whatever you may believe to be a good communication idea, you should always try to check whether or not it actually works! As Stockwell (1985) stressed, the bottom line is that people understand one another and agree on a decision.

A number of specific methods for enhancing the effectiveness of communication have been developed. These are mostly derived from direct work, but they apply with equal strength when one is communicating with a mediator.

Listen carefully

Active attention to verbal and nonverbal cues is an obvious guideline, but one which is regularly broken. Bernstein and Halaszyn (1989) suggest that *paraphrasing* is a useful check on your active listening. This is based on repeating the other person's ideas back to them in your own words. An example would be checking whether the carer of an elderly person said that they were finding their dependent's wandering to be a greater source of stress than their memory failings. Additionally, paraphrasing can elicit more useful information, such as 'Yes, but it's not just wandering, it's the risk of hurting herself that bothers me most of all'.

A second test you can perform is *perception checking*. This involves finding out whether the mediator is actually feeling what you think they are feeling. To continue the example, it would be saying something like: 'I sense that you are partly anxious and partly angry about your mother's wandering'.

There are also nonverbal signs of active listening, such as eye contact, note-taking and nodding. In contrast, other cues such as fidgeting and restlessness, would tend to suggest inattention.

Exercise 8.1: Active listening

As an exercise in active listening, try to discern a few key messages which a colleague is conveying to you. If possible, try to place them in order of importance. This includes verbal and nonverbal information, as well as primary and secondary messages. Once you have assessed these messages, check them out with your colleague, trying to explain why you decided that these were important (especially the secondary messages). This can be done in the context of a case discussion.

To illustrate, your colleague might describe a client who is depressed and experiencing sleep disturbance, restlessness and a sense of helplessness about their life. While describing these features your colleague may indicate exasperation or a sense of futility in working with this client. This might be conveyed by a resigned tone and a lack of interest or ideas about the client.

Speak carefully

The content and form of our speech are also obvious factors in communication. Less apparent are such things as the choice or precision of the language we use. These will influence not only whether the primary message is received ('fuzzy' words such as 'aggression' may hamper communication) but also whether other messages are conveyed. Thus, if we referred to the carer above as 'overprotective', or 'anxious', we would convey a different message than if we said she was 'concerned' or 'thoughtful'. While all these terms may be based on exactly the same information about the carer, the speaker has interpreted the information in such a way as to convey an unfavourable or favourable picture of her. This would be secondary communication, in contrast to the primary one which focused on whether the elderly person wandered or had short-term memory problems. Similarly, jargon may be used to try and convey expertise.

With regard to the form of our communications, Ley's (1977) famous research work on doctor–patient communication has highlighted the importance of the following ways of talking, when trying to gain compliance:

- be friendly rather than businesslike
- engage in at least some conversation which is not directly connected with the problem
- discover the mediator's expectations and try to explain why these may be realistic or unrealistic
- discuss the mediator's concerns and attempt to allay these
- give information as well as asking questions.

Although these guidelines may appear obvious and straightforward, attempts to implement indirect therapy programmes suggest a need for the provision of considerable structure for the therapist. To illustrate, in a family therapy approach to schizophrenia, reading materials are designed to help guide discussions between therapist and the schizophrenic person's family. In turn, these are designed to modify the expressed emotion (EE) communicated by the family, although reading and discussion are usually supplemented by the role playing of low EE forms of communication with the dependent person (see, for example, Bennun and Lucas, 1990).

Exercise 8.2: The use of adjectives

As an exercise in studying speech, make a written note of all the adjectives used by your colleagues to describe carers or clients, perhaps during a case review, or from the care plan. Try to categorise each adjective in terms of the emotional value you perceive it as having, using the categories 'positive', 'neutral' and 'negative'. If, for example, a carer is described as 'overconcerned' you might categorise this as negative, whereas the adjective 'protective' might seem positive to you.

Write carefully

In addition, when the communication is in written form, it generally helps to provide simple, unambiguous messages (jargon or technical terms should be avoided). Research also suggests that a *primacy effect* is often present, meaning that people tend to remember those bits of information that are given at the beginning of a message.

An example of the use of written communications is someone working with a co-therapist in relation to a group for depressed clients. A generally useful model has been provided by Hops (1976), based on work with couples between whom communication has gone awry. Step One is pinpointing what is to be done in the group sessions. This might include not just the detailed content, but also writing down who will do what and for how long. The result should be a precise, detailed programme. Step Two entails checking that you and the co-therapist agree about the programme. This may take the form of a typed memo or a more detailed handwritten (but photocopied) note. By doing so the other party has an opportunity to compare notes and to move towards an agreed programme.

Step Three may involve some further exchanges if any disagreement remains. These might suggest other ways of organising the group, perhaps negotiating new ideas. Lastly, Hops (1976) suggests that contracting may be helpful, especially if the preceding steps are not working. This would specify who would do what, dependent upon certain conditions. A conventional example would be for the co-therapists to contract with an agency to provide the group therapy in exchange for a fee or some form of reciprocation (for example, use of the agency's rooms for some direct work).

Although writing things down usually feels like an unnecessary burden at the time, my own experience has confirmed that with hindsight it is a very good investment of time and effort, particularly in indirect work. Should you have doubts about this, you can assess the utility of different written communications in the following exercise.

Exercise 8.3: Communication

Next time you are in a meeting, compare notes on what was agreed with a colleague. Independently note down such details as: What was agreed? Who would do what? By when? In order to achieve what outcome? In addition to comparing your own notes also take account of the minutes from the meeting (especially the 'Action' column) and the continued discussion of the matter at the next meeting. I would be surprised if there were not one or two clear disagreements on these points somewhere along the communication chain. Whether or not there are disagreements, compare the meeting or the notes against the guidelines here (was there any 'pinpointing'? Was an explicit agreement reached?).

A case study

I met a team leader for Community Psychiatric Nurses to discuss indirect work. As he is partly based in a new community mental health centre and partly covers a geographic 'patch', I thought that he would be able to provide good examples of indirect work. Thus, like some earlier case studies, this one considers examples drawn from several areas of one nurse's work.

In terms of communication, the team leader highlighted the importance of relationships between the CPN and carers (or other professionals) as a critical factor. When he had established a good relationship, communication could become more open and influential. For example, he believed that one of his clients was able to tell him things because he had earned her trust, and also he represented a relatively 'non-threatening' professional (that is, not exercising any statutory powers over the client in this instance of child abuse). He felt that he could obtain the best possible service for his clients from other professionals when there already existed between them a relationship based on reciprocity and the free expression of viewpoints.

When working indirectly, this CPN used a range of communication mediums, including one-to-one meetings, phone conversations and letters. These were employed as appropriate, generally becoming more formal if the message was not achieving its aim. As a rule, he used written communications to record what had been said, to summarise his observations, and to clearly state the action that he felt was required. In one example, he felt that a case conference was necessary but that the social worker concerned was procrastinating. He therefore moved from phone calls to sending a letter, which clearly set out his case for holding the conference. This was copied to all other interested parties, including the social worker's manager. This course of action led to the case conference he had sought, nicely illustrating the earlier point that the effectiveness of any communication should be judged by its results.

While this kind of action can undermine the relationship between people, the CPN believed that clear and sometimes forceful communication of this kind is part of being professional. He thinks that, in general, nurses have shrunk back from making assertive observations about clients' difficulties, or from advocating appropriate care, leaving these activities to other disciplines. He was therefore communicating a second kind of message in this example, namely that nurses have the right to insist on being heard! This important dimension of communication shows that the way in which we present our message will signal things about the sender, sometimes referred to as *meta communication*.

Teaching and training

Accounts of the mental health nurse's role tend to stress direct work, with little attention being paid to indirect activities such as teaching or training. Cormack's (1983) review does not mention these activities explicitly, although his data, based on a sample of over 4,000 'critical incidents', do suggest an educative role. For example, informing relatives about the treatment of an illness and enabling them to play an active part in care are presumably based on some form of 'teaching'. More directly, he noted nearly 100 incidents when the psychiatric nurses in his large study taught, counselled or orientated staff. My dictionary defines teaching as 'showing, directing, guiding and counselling', which suggests that nurses may be educating in a diverse range of ways, direct *and* indirect. For instance the nurse's perspective on a client presented in a case review or multidisciplinary team meeting may well educate others, although not presented as formal teaching. Co-therapy and general discussion of clients and their care are other illustrations of potentially educational interactions between nurses and other staff or carers. Perhaps it is the informal nature of these exchanges which leads to the lack of emphasis on teaching in the nurse's role.

There do appear to be good grounds for emphasising teaching as a way of influencing the work of mediators. The arguments would be based on the fact of working closely together, and the need for at least part of the contact time to be based on education, even if it is purely concerned with delimiting the nurse's role to a mediator. More powerfully, it would be based on the advantages of teaching, and particularly of training, as a way of influencing how other people work. This relates to the arguments advanced earlier in favour of the triadic model (for example, effectiveness and efficiency). Training, in turn, concerns practical instruction, and can be distinguished from teaching by such features as its methods and goals. Thus, while the teacher seeks to educate people to think for themselves, the trainer prepares people to practise a specific skill. So while one is broadranging and concerned with developing a challenging way of thinking about things, the other focuses on imparting the accepted approach to things, almost a 'master–apprentice' relationship.

However, in practice, these potentially distinguishable activities are often blended, particularly in applied settings such as hospitals. Workshops, although typically a training endeavour, may include significant educational goals and methods. Additionally, the way that we learn can blur the distinctions still further, as an ancient Chinese proverb put it:

> I hear and I forget
> I see and I remember
> I do and I understand

Cormack's (1983) study suggests that nurses do a great deal of informal teaching and training, by providing opportunities to talk, offering explanations, encouraging understanding and in facilitating independence. At one level these may seem to be simply elements of 'caring', but at another they indicate an educational emphasis, helping people to learn and change. This would apply in indirect as well as direct work, as indicated by the earlier examples of teamwork and case reviews.

Teaching carers

Having suggested that much direct and indirect nursing work may fundamentally be teaching and training, let me now consider an example of each in some detail. Firstly I would like to focus on teaching, particularly as a specific element in interventions with carers of elderly people. As the study by Bennum and Lucas (1990) indicated, family therapy for people with schizophrenia is based on a package including reading material and discussion. In the case of the carers of elderly people, there is a considerable history of educational effort. This follows from the relatives' unawareness of some of the basic facts of their dependent's condition. By providing this information in a structured way, nurses can help to educate carers about such conditions as a dementia and thereby help to alter their attitudes and behaviour towards the elderly person. Information on how other carers cope and on the available help may also be useful. In addition to information on dementia and resources, nurses can participate in support groups by helping carers to learn better ways of nursing their dependent person at home. Woods and Britton (1985) have reviewed research, which shows that this educational component was preferred by carers to training in forms of self-help.

As an example of this research, consider a study conducted by Greene and Monahan (1987) in the USA, in which carers of elderly family members received support and education from a social worker and a community health nurse. The carers attended eight weekly two-hour sessions, each one including the following components:

- *group discussion*: this was intended to assist carers to deal with negative feelings arising from caregiving and to overcome their sense of isolation. Successful ways of solving caring problems were elicited and emphasised;

- *education*: a curriculum of talks was organised to address useful ideas and techniques, such as how to lift, move and bathe the dependent elderly person. The programme also included information on the ageing process and the course of dementia;

- *relaxation*: carers were taught various methods for achieving a state of calm and a composed state of mind, including the use of imagery and progressive muscular relaxation.

Greene and Monahan found that this package of support and education reduced the likelihood that the elderly dependent person would require institutional care. They calculated that this represented a saving of one-third of a million dollars for their sample of 36 dependent people, over the six month period of the research.

Similarly positive outcomes from teaching interventions have been reported by Lovett and Gallagher (1988), who evaluated the impact of a 'coping skills' package for family caregivers on their depression and morale. Two different teaching packages of 10 two-hour session were compared. The first focused on the carer's capacity to enhance their mood. This was pursued by teaching the carers to monitor and increasingly control their mood and their 'pleasant events'. The second package entailed a problem-solving approach. Carers were taught to specify problems, 'brainstorm' potential solutions, analyse the pros and

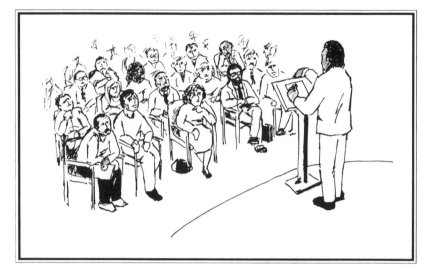

Teaching is an important but underemphasised aspect of nursing

cons of these, implement the selected solution and then evaluate the outcome. Lovett and Gallagher found that carers who received both packages had lower levels of depression and higher morale than carers assigned to a waiting list condition.

The value of a teaching role has also been demonstrated with other client groups, in both general and psychiatric nursing. Wallace (1986), for instance, showed that an information booklet given to women undergoing minor gynaecological surgery helped to increase their knowledge while reducing their anxieties and facilitating a faster recovery. Closer to mental health nursing, problem drinkers receiving a self-help manual were better at controlling their drinking than those receiving general advice and information (Heather *et al.* (1987)). Taken together, these studies indicate that teaching can play a valuable role as an indirect form of nursing practice.

Training staff

As previously suggested, training has by definition less of an educational emphasis. In conducting training, the nurse is explicitly shaping the work behaviour of others towards practical objectives, such as improved communication with clients. Characteristically, the trainer draws on a body of knowledge. This knowledge base is then organised in such a way that trainees can learn to apply it to their own work. This in turn involves determining the content and methods of the training event, in the same way as the carers received their teaching in the form of a 'package'. I will now illustrate these points by detailed reference to an in-service training workshop provided to nurses in psychiatric rehabilitation (Milne *et al.*, 1985). The workshop was led by various professionals, including psychiatrists, psychologists and nurses.

The 'core course' in behaviour therapy

In this example, the course content and methods were derived from prior research in behaviour therapy and skills training. Thus the topics were drawn from existing studies of nurse training in this area, allied to the practical objectives of the workshop. These dictated that we cover such things as observational methods of recording client behaviour and behavioural strategies for altering this behaviour (especially operant and classical conditioning techniques). These topics were organised in a sequence of steps, each one building on its predecessors. The whole course lasted one week.

Similarly, the workshop methods reflected what was known about facilitating skill and knowledge acquisition. The *structured learning format* was employed throughout the workshop. This consisted of a combination of teaching methods, including lectures, reading, modelling and practical exercises with feedback.

The ultimate aim of the 'core course' workshop was to help nurses to plan and conduct their individual care plans. Preliminary aims were to increase their skills and knowledge in behaviour therapy. We evaluated the workshop in these and other areas, obtaining positive findings. In terms of knowledge, the nurses obtained a higher score on a multiple choice questionnaire following the workshop. They also did much better on measures of skill, including video-presented observation tasks in the classroom; and in work with their own clients on their wards (these are considered in more detail in Chapter 10).

However, while the evaluations of knowledge and skill were favourable, the workshop did not appear to increase the proportion of care plans conducted on the wards by these nurses. We therefore revised the core course, altering it from a 'classroom' based to a 'client-centred' format. This meant that during the practical phase of the structured learning format, we encouraged nurses to work with a selected client on their ward, rather than role-play. This inevitably took up more time, but we were able to accommodate this within the one week period by reducing the number of learning steps within the workshops.

Training and innovation

As a result of this change, a far higher proportion of care plans were implemented, with an increase from 26 per cent to 75 per cent. This illustrates how evaluation can guide the organisation of training events so that practical aims are achieved. It also shows that workshops can be relatively ineffective, at least when judged in term of changes in work behaviour or client benefit. Indeed, the history of training generally is one peppered with examples of fruitless effort. In a famous article, Georgiades and Phillimore (1975) reviewed the effectiveness of training ventures, concluding that they were not successful as a means of innovating services. Indeed, they found evidence that training could actually make matters worse, by making people more aware of the shortcomings of their current methods. They argued that the crucial factor determining the success of training was the 'back home environment'. In the case of psychiatric nurses, this might be the reaction of colleagues or clients to any ideas gathered from a workshop. If their reaction to innovative methods is positive, then the training can be applied to good effect. In this sense, training is often regarded as a necessary but insufficient basis for improving the quality of care. To be sufficient, the training has to be combined with a supportive work environment. For this reason, trainers will sometimes negotiate adequate managerial support before they agree to undertake any training. For the core course, the nurses who had received the training and gone on to make use of it stated that the support of their colleagues (including that of their managers) had been a critical factor, as had the success of the behavioural methods carried out with their clients.

The case study

To return to the present case study, like Cormack's (1983) sample, the CPN team leader had also been involved in a diverse range of teaching activities, from educating to training. On the educational side, he had contributed to teaching sessions for Age Concern care attendants who provided a carer support scheme, offering a nurse's view of the problems associated with dementia. He had also spent a day with student nurses addressing basic assumptions about work in the community. Similar teaching efforts had been directed at children in the local school and at interested members of the public attending a drop-in centre.

Moving to 'training', he had taken opportunities in case conferences to challenge prevailing beliefs and assumptions, such as the tendency for hospital-based staff to work towards goals which exceeded the level of functioning accepted in the client's home context. In case conferences he had been able to suggest new techniques, such as adopting family therapy approaches with elderly people and their families. Moving closer still to training, he had facilitated group work on the topic of bereavement and had contributed to the ENB course on 'Care of the Elderly'.

Social support interventions

The role of social support as a complement to personal coping strategies in dealing with life stressors has been outlined in Chapters 1 and 2 in Niven and Robinson (1993). Social support is evidently an important element in mental health, so it follows that nurses should be concerned with facilitating it. Working directly with a client often involves both analysis of, and intervention in, social support, in such areas as social skills training or encouraging the client to engage in antidepressive activities. In addition, a nurse might work indirectly on social support, so that potential or long-standing clients receive the best possible levels of support from those around them or from community settings.

A good illustration of such indirect social support work was provided by the CPN whose work represents the case study in this chapter. He has been involved with a health promotion project based in a council house, which was intended to provide advice and support to the people who lived on the estate. As these included a number of clients from his caseload, he had good reason to help the project achieve its objectives. This he did by supervising the direct work of the volunteers and the development worker who ran the project. He also offered general support and his own contributions in the form of some direct work and a group session on benzodiazepine withdrawal. In addition, the nurse was a member of the steering group, helping to plan the effective running of the project.

This example illustrates a blend of socially supportive activities by a mental health nurse. However, nurses can also work indirectly to improve social support by giving information, emotional support or practical assistance, as I will illustrate.

Informational support

Much useful social support work goes on at the level of the mediator, as discussed earlier in the context of teaching carers of the elderly about dementia. As noted at that stage, giving information can be a simple yet powerful form of indirect help. In addition, nurses can work at the social, or organisational, level, providing information to those who are responsible for running organisations such as schools, shops or factories. The most obvious form this might take is mental health education or promotion, by providing talks or leaflets. Another way of conveying information to the general public is by having displays at fairs and exhibitions. At the time of writing, the local CPN service has had a stand at the recent town fair, where they gave out leaflets with information on their service. Such efforts can help to prevent mental

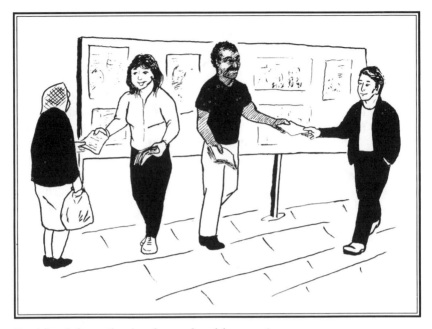

Providing information is a form of social support

health problems, or help those who have difficulties to locate the most appropriate service.

Professionals can also contribute to mental health promotion by working with the media in radio phone-in programmes or articles in local newspapers. In one study of radio phone-in programmes, Bouthoutsos *et al.* (1986) found that half of their large sample of adults had listened to programmes concerned with advice and information about human relationships. They had found these helpful and educational, although some speculated that these programmes might be harmful. The small amount of evidence available from this study indicated that there was no adverse change in the listeners' wellbeing, even though quite a high proportion had followed the advice they received. As half of the sample reported having been in therapy, there is a clear link to direct work, as in the earlier case study example of the health education project. Another link is the effect attributed by the sample to listening to the programmes. Apparently this can help family communication, strengthen the sense of 'community' and reduce anxieties about coping with stressors.

Emotional support

The CPN team leader's work with the health education project illustrated a non-specific support role for the CPN in helping volunteers to provide counselling. Based on a review of the literature, Nolan and Grant (1989) delineated four types of help provided by the professional to the carer. These were information giving, skills training, emotional support and respite care. The emotional support was construed at a number of levels:

- recognising and valuing the carer's work
- talking over the problems of caring
- recognising and dealing with a number of emotions (for example, guilt, anger, depression)
- setting limits on the care given by the carer
- negotiating responsibilities with their dependent

Nolan and Grant (1989) went on to conduct a postal survey of carers, finding that they reported major deficiencies in the four main areas listed. They saw emotional support as being the area most in need of the professionals' attention. For example, being valued and appreciated for their efforts was a crucial determinant of carer satisfaction. Moreover, in its absence, the carer's stress was higher. Because of such findings, these authors argued that professionals should give much more attention to the provision of emotional support to carers. To enable this, they put forward a practice model (based on stress and adaptation) and proposed changes in the education of nurses.

Practical support

An interesting paper by Maton (1989) draws a helpful distinction between three levels of work in social support carried out by mental health professionals. These are the *individual* (for example, bolstering support-elicitation skills), *interpersonal* (as in providing practical support to someone), and *organisational*. The latter refers to such phenomena as a sense of belonging, or community, and social integration in the context of social settings (for example, neighbourhoods, work, school). Maton (1989) reports three studies at this organisational level, where attention was directed at factors in the settings that facilitated support. He considered religious congregations, mutual help groups and centres for old people, concluding that they each served to buffer the members from stress in distinctive ways. Church-going appeared to provide meaning, hope and a world view; the mutual help group fostered coping skills, information-sharing and the opportunity to help others; while the centres provided supportive relationships, activities and practical help.

The evidence to date on the benefits to mental health of such support is inconclusive, as the few studies reported tend to rely on simple correlational methods. These make cause–effect interpretations impossible. However, evidence from the individual and interpersonal levels is more decisive, indicating a definite role for social support. On the assumption that these findings will be obtained at the organisational level, nurses may usefully work on promoting self-help groups and even on facilitating social support in larger or less familiar community settings, such as churches and centres.

In terms of practical support for groups, nurses can help by locating suitable venues; advertising and recruiting members; recruiting and selecting the volunteers to lead the groups; organising transport, equipment and materials (such as self-help booklets and relaxation tapes); and they can 'enable' the whole process by organising crèches or respite care for members who would otherwise be unable to attend. Similar kinds of practical help might be arranged in relation to organisational work.

Summary

Working indirectly raises special challenges and opportunities for nurses, ones which seem inevitable in relation to community care. Work in the community entails larger numbers of clients, more diffuse social networks and a wider range of ways of maintaining mental health, therefore requiring the nurse to consider new work practices. Generally labelled as indirect *methods in this chapter, they include the challenge of effective communication and the opportunities for social support work. But indirect work can also apply with equal strength to the traditional hospital setting, as in the roles of educator and trainer. I argue that such indirect work is especially important in relation to the impact, effectiveness and efficiency of a service. The case study material generates an additional argument. This is the way in which indirect work aids analysis of 'the problem': examination of health education projects and other similar projects helps in the conceptualisation of mental health, leading to ideas for revised practice.*

Indirect work subsumes a vast range of activities, and only the more obvious examples have been discussed in this chapter. Another common example is the role of research and evaluation, to which I will turn next.

Questions for further consideration

1 Although indirect work has some obvious advantages, many clinicians shy away from it. What reasons can you provide for this?
2 How might you determine the appropriate balance between direct

and indirect work? (It may help to consider this in relation to a specific ward or role.)

3 Nurses who work through mediators such as carers might be accused by their more traditional colleagues of diluting, distorting or even destroying their role. How might one weigh up these accusations?

4 In relation to a ward you know well, how might communication be improved? Consider the needs of 'sender', 'medium' and 'receiver' separately.

5 Imagine that you are a CPN team leader concerned about poor communication skills amongst your colleagues. Taking account of the available guidelines, how might this problem be tackled?

6 Teaching and training work need to be adapted in order to take account of the most appropriate learning methods to achieve objectives. How would you run a workshop which was intended to alter nurses' attitudes towards the elderly? (You may find it helpful to draw on your own learning experiences as a student.)

References

Bennun, I. and Lucas, R. (1990). Using the partner in the psychosocial treatment of schizophrenia: a multiple single case design. *British Journal of Clinical Psychology, 29*, 185–192.

Bernstein, G. S. (1984). Training of behaviour change agents. In R. M. Eisler and P. M. Miller (Eds) *Progress in Behaviour Modification* (Volume 17) New York: Academic Press.

Bernstein, G. S. and Halaszyn, J. A. (1989) *'Human Services? . . . That must be so rewarding.'* London: Paul Brookes.

Bochner, S. (1983). Doctors, patients and their cultures. In D. Pendleton and J. Hasler, *Doctor–Patient Communication.* London: Academic Press.

Bouhoutsos, J. C., Goodchilds, J. D. and Huddy, L. (1986). Media psychology: an empirical study of radio call-in psychology programmes. *Professional Psychology: Research and Practice, 17*, 408–414.

Cormack, D. F. S. (1983). *Psychiatric Nursing Described.* Edinburgh: Churchill Livingstone.

Georgiades, N. J. and Phillimore, L. (1975). The myth of the hero-innovator and alternative strategies for organisational change. In C. C. Kiernan and F. P. Woodford (Eds) *Behaviour Modification with the Severely Retarded.* New York: Associated Scientific Publishers.

Goldberg, D. and Huxley, P. (1980). *Mental Illness in the Community.* London: Tavistock.

Greene, V. L. and Monahan, D. J. (1987). The effect of a professionally guided caregiver support and education group on institutionalisation of care receivers. *The Gerontologist, 27*, 716–721.

Heather, N., Robertson, I., MacPherson, B., Allsop, S. and Fulton, A. (1987). Effectiveness of a controlled drinking self-help manual: one year follow-up results. *British Journal of Clinical Psychology, 26*, 279–287.

Hops, H. (1976). Behaviour treatment of marital problems. In W. E. Craighead, A. E. Kazdin and M. S. Mahoney (Eds) *Behaviour Modification.* Boston: Houghton Mifflin.

Johnston, M. (1982). Recognition of patients' worries by nurses and by other patients. *British Journal of Clinical Psychology, 21*, 255–261.

Ley, P. (1977). Psychological research on doctor–patient communication. In S. J. Rachman (Ed.) *Advances in Medical Psychology.* Oxford: Pergamon Press.

Lovett, S. and Gallagher, D. (1988). Psychoeducational interventions for family caregivers: preliminary efficacy data. *Behaviour Therapy, 19*, 321–330.

Maton, K. I. (1989). Community settings as buffers of life stress? Highly supportive churches, mutual help groups and senior centres. *American Journal of Community Psychology, 17*, 203–232.

Milne, D. L., Burdett, C. and Conway, P. (1985). Review and replications of a core course in behaviour therapy for psychiatric nurses. *Journal of Advanced Nursing, 10*, 137–148.

Niven, N. (1989). *Health Psychology: An introduction for nurses and other health care professionals.* Edinburgh: Churchill-Livingstone.

Niven, N., and Robinson, J. (1993). *The Psychology of Nursing Care: A foundation text.* Leicester: BPS Books (The British Psychological Society) and London: Macmillan.

Nolan, M. R. and Grant, G. (1989). Addressing the needs of informal carers: a neglected area of nursing practice. *Journal of Advanced Nursing, 14*, 950–961.

Sayal, S. (1990). Black women and mental health. *The Psychologist, 3*, 24–27.

Shepherd, M., Cooper, B., Brown, A. C. and Katton, G. (1966). *Psychiatric Illness in General Practice.* London: Oxford University Press.

Stockwell, F. (1985). *The Nursing Process in Psychiatric Nursing.* London: Croom Helm.

Tomlinson, A. (1985). The use of experimental methods in teaching inter-personal skills to nurses. In C. Kagan (Ed.) *Interpersonal Skills in Nursing.* London: Croom Helm.

Wallace, L. M. (1986). Communication variables in the design of pre-surgical preparatory information. *British Journal of Clinical Psychology, 25*, 111–118.

Woods, R. T. and Britton, P. G. (1985). *Clinical Psychology with the Elderly.* London: Routledge.

Further reading

Egan, G. (1986). *The Skilled Helper.* Monterey: Brooks/Cole.
A classic text which is interesting for at least two reasons. Firstly, Egan emphasises a clear, simple problem-solving framework throughout, one that is strikingly similar to the nursing process (that is, it consists of problem definition, goal development and action). Secondly, there are two chapters devoted to communication, specifically 'attending and listening', and 'empathy and probing'.

Foster, M. C. and Mayall, B. (1990). Health Visitors as Educators. *Journal of Advanced Nursing, 15*, 286–292.
This paper sets out four models for health education and reports a study of staff and client perceptions of child health care. The Health Visitor's initial training as a nurse represents a common base with mental health nursing, and, as they discuss, tends to lead to the preference of a 'persuasive' model of health education.

Slater, J. (1990). Effecting personal effectiveness: assertiveness training for nurses. *Journal of Advanced Nursing, 15*, 337–356.
This paper offers some interesting explanations of the unassertive nurse and outlines a 'personal effectiveness' workshop designed to rectify matters.

Ward, M. F. (1985). *The Nursing Process in Psychiatry*. Edinburgh: Churchill Livingstone.
A practical book which includes a section on the nursing process in the community. Here you will find suggestions on liaison between hospital and community (another form of 'communication'), comments on the education of nurses, and ideas on developing the nursing role in the community (for example, 'crisis intervention' work).

SECTION FIVE
Evaluation

9 *Introduction to evaluation*

Evaluation is a judgement of the extent to which nursing care plans (or services) achieve their goals. It therefore represents the final element of the nursing process as a problem-solving strategy. Like the other three elements, evaluation is a necessary but insufficient basis for problem-solving. In addition to its place in problem-solving, evaluation has grown in importance with the emphasis on quality in mental health services; 'quality assurance' and 'quality standards' are based on evaluation.

Although evaluation holds this important position, it tends to be more often promised than practised. This seems to be due to its association with various unpleasant manifestations of evaluation, such as examinations, and to its relatively minor emphasis in health care practice. The major emphasis appears to be given to implementation methods with their positive connotations of help-giving. This bias away from evaluation is a pity since, when construed in terms of 'feedback', evaluation has a very positive contribution to make. There are many ways in which evaluation can serve this useful feedback function. The range may not parallel the numerous implementation options, but it holds considerable scope for applying interesting and feasible methods.

This chapter is intended to demonstrate the rewards of evaluation, especially in relation to your direct work with clients, while the next chapter will consider the evaluation of indirect work. However, as you will see, the principles and methods of evaluation apply equally to direct and indirect work.

In outlining these rewards, I will start by examining the nature of evaluation. I will do this by comparing it with research, before describing the different types of evaluation. The type of most interest to health care professionals is *outcome* evaluation, the determination of the impact or effectiveness of care plans. However, the other forms of evaluation are complementary and when combined, they tend to yield a more accurate picture of a care programme. For this reason I will also consider the evaluation of *process*, *efficiency* and *acceptability*, advocating a broad approach.

The remaining section deals with evaluation procedures. This is relatively straightforward, insofar as the nursing process already requires that you incorporate at least two of the main steps – goal setting and intervention.

What is 'evaluation'?

In ordinary language, 'evaluation' is the judgement of how much something is worth. In health care it tends to be defined as the extent to which the goals of a service are achieved. When combined with rigorous methods of data-gathering, it is often referred to as *service evaluation* or *evaluative research*, although there are many closely related terms (for example action, applied or field research). The defining characteristics of service evaluation are as follows (Milne, 1987):

- identifying and defining goals;
- analysing problems which the service must face;
- describing and standardising the service;
- measuring the amount of change that occurs;
- determining by research methods the extent to which change is attributable to the service; and
- assessing the relative effectiveness of modified services.

These characteristics distinguish evaluation from 'pure' or 'laboratory' research. For example, research is not primarily concerned with practical problems and solutions, but rather with theory development. *Table 9.1* lists some of these distinctions, although it should be realised that this is a rather simplified way of considering what are basically two different forms of research.

As *Table 9.1* shows, these two kinds of research differ on at least eleven counts. In reviewing evaluation in nursing, Luker (1981) defined it as 'applied research where the major aim is not the generation of new knowledge but the study of the application of existing knowledge' (p87). This perhaps best represents Factor 1 in *Table 9.1*, suggesting that there are several other ways of defining evaluation. Amongst these are its restriction to socially important phenomena (for example, clients and carers). Also, evaluation is intended to improve practical matters within a specific setting, whereas research is concerned with general truths. For these kinds of reasons, journals tend to be associated with one or other of these traditions. Those journals which are intended to address practical issues in relation to health care professionals will therefore tend to focus on evaluation, whereas the more specific research journals will deal with a wide range of issues considered to be of theoretical importance.

Exercise 9.1: Categorising journals as research or evaluation focused
As an exercise, try to locate two journals in your library, one representing 'research' (for example, the *British Medical Journal*), the other 'evaluation'

(for example, the *Journal of Advanced Nursing*). Use the criteria in *Table 9.1* in order to make this categorisation. Try to note one or two articles from each of these journals which deviate from the criteria in *Table 9.1*. For example, you may find an article in a research journal with a very practical topic and findings; or an evaluation journal article with good scientific standards. Having studied the contents of these two kinds of journal, what general distinctions from *Table 9.1* would you feel able to draw? Can you add any other distinctions?

Table 9.1 *Some of the typical distinctions drawn between evaluation and research (compiled from Popham, 1975; Suchman, 1967)*

Factor	Research	Evaluation
1. Purpose of research	To build theories and improve understanding	To make decisions and improve programmes
2. Applicability of findings	Widely applicable	Results only directly relevant to same programme and setting
3. Value of research	To establish 'truth'	To improve worth of programme
4. Measurement	Standardised instruments; rigorous scientific standards essential (for example randomisation)	Ragbag of measuring tools; control very difficult to achieve; scientific standards desirable
5. Topics	Anything	Socially important phenomena
6. Judgement	Eschewed	Integral
7. Research consumers	Secondary, not identified	Primary
8. Politics	An improper consideration	A necessary and important consideration
9. Replicability	Important hallmarks	Neither important nor possible
10. Setting	Not treated as significant; highly controlled	Essential aspect; control very limited
11. Publication	Major academic goal of research	Uncommon and secondary

Blurring the distinctions

In practice it is becoming increasingly difficult to make these kinds of distinctions. This seems to be due largely to the increasingly sophisticated research methods used in evaluation. A good example of this, the case study, will be considered shortly. However, it is worth noting that a great majority of service evaluations are never published in any kind of journal, as they tend to be poorly controlled or unsophisticated in some other aspect indicated in *Table 9.1*. This is not to say that they necessarily represent bad professional practice, since the information from the evaluation may still provide a better basis for decision-making than the more common judgemental basis. Indeed, an evaluation might be very rigorous from a scientific standpoint, but as it deals with a highly local or much researched topic, such as needs assessment with elderly people, it will not merit publication.

Different types of evaluation

Following the impressive work of Suchman (1967), five different kinds of evaluation focus will be outlined. They are *outcome, effort, process, efficiency* and *acceptability*. These are complementary aspects of a service, and ideally an evaluation should consider all five of them. Suchman considered such a combination to be an 'ultimate' evaluation. Although desirable, it is rare enough to come across process–outcome evaluations, far less 'ultimate' or total ones. This is not to suggest that those carrying out small-scale, local evaluations should be deterred from considering the 'ultimate' combination of topics, since it is quite feasible to gather some information under four of these headings but to focus on a fifth. A common example would be where the focus is on outcome evaluation, while the collation of readily available information on some of the remaining headings, such as the number of staff providing a service, would represent a complementary 'effort' evaluation. Just as evaluation is a necessary but insufficient basis for a problem-solving model (as in the nursing process), so each of these five topics is a necessary but insufficient basis for evaluation. Only the ultimate evaluation is sufficient.

Outcome evaluation

Two kinds of outcome evaluation have been distinguished by Suchman (1967). The first concerns the effect of care plans on individual clients, for example in reducing their incontinence, or increasing their independence. A second type of outcome evaluation is the impact that this work has on these kinds of problems throughout a community. In other words, a marvellous but labour-intensive therapy could be 100 per cent effective but have little impact, as it can only be provided to a very small proportion of those who would benefit. Comprehensive mental health services have to balance their *effectiveness* against their *impact*, developing relatively easily administered but adequately effective forms of intervention. The use of self-help booklets, social support networks and the media are possible options in this regard, as discussed in Chapter 8.

Outcome evaluations, whether of effectiveness or impact, lie at the very heart of evaluation. They cover the most important things anyone would want to know about a therapy or a service, and essentially deal with the questions: 'Does it work?' 'How well?'; 'For whom?' If something does not work, people are unlikely to be interested in the effort, process, or any other aspect of the intervention. Therefore, only after the generation of some good results do we tend to start thinking about these secondary forms of evaluation. It is for this reason that I have started with this type of evaluation.

Effectiveness can also be usefully subdivided into two forms. One form concerns the question of whether a client has improved or not. Very small improvements on a number of evaluation measures (for example, a battery of questionnaires and ratings) can yield a statistically significant difference between a client's score on these measures before and after a care plan. It is then tempting to conclude that the client is 'better'. The second form of effectiveness evaluation disregards the statistical solution in favour of *clinical significance* (Barlow *et al.*, 1984). As the term suggests, this judges effectiveness in terms of sufficient change to produce an important improvement in a client's functioning, in the sense that the client is able to do something that he or she could not do prior to the care plan. The general term for the clinical significance type of evaluation is *goal-attainment*. It depends on establishing a baseline (pre-intervention) measure of the client's functioning and clarifying relevant goals, so this form of evaluation is perhaps closest to the nursing process.

As an illustration of a goal-attainment evaluation, consider a case study provided by Stanley (1984). He used the *Goal Attainment Scale* to establish some appropriate goals for a client in the psychiatric rehabilitation sector of a large hospital. These included cooking breakfast, attending social events and shaving. Each goal was broken down into five levels, from much less than expected (-2) to much more than expected ($+2$), and each goal was also assigned a weighting to take account of its relative importance. Once progress with such a care plan has been reviewed, it is possible to evaluate this progress in a systematic way by the use of a formula.

Illustrations of the 'statistical significance' form of effectiveness evaluation are much more common, as illustrated by the questionnaires, ratings and observations used to evaluate the two day hospitals mentioned earlier (Milne, 1984). Barker (1987) provides a review of the kind of client problems and the evaluative measures used in psychiatric nursing. One of his examples, based on reductions in medication use, illustrates how a variety of variables may serve in an effectiveness evaluation.

Before leaving this form of evaluation, I should mention that *statistical* significance and *clinical* significance are not necessarily distinct. Some questionnaires, for example, allow the evaluator to relate the score achieved by a client to that achieved by defined groups (norms), as in the *Clifton Assessment Procedures for the Elderly (CAPE*; Pattie, 1981). This can lead to highly practical conclusions, such as the type of residential care that is appropriate for that client.

However, not all changes in mental health nursing lend themselves to measurement, although they may be of great significance. It is necessary to recognise that there is considerable doubt in some quarters that mental health outcomes can be measured, far less form the basis of an evaluation. For instance Strupp (1973) has listed 15 common 'lessons' or outcomes associated with analytically-orientated therapy. In essence these are new beliefs or insights about the self and about others, held by the client with different levels of conviction following therapy. *Table 9.2* summarises some of these lessons. The therapist's, or client's judgements about the extent to which these sorts of lessons were learned would normally serve as the outcome evaluation, although not usually formalised in this way.

Turning to impact, it is rare to find studies which have considered the extent to which a therapy or service has benefited a community. Such a study would, for instance, indicate the proportion of suitable people who had been provided with the service, and with what results. That is, it builds on an evaluation of effectiveness by asking how widespread the effects are of a service.

One of these rare examples of impact evaluation has been provided by Falloon *et al.* (1987). Their Buckinghamshire project entailed a home-based mental health service for a community of some 40,000 people, implemented through the existing health and social agencies. Teams of four to five nurses received a two-year-long training programme led by a senior nurse therapist. The project entailed rapid consultation with clients (that is, within 24 hours), and the use of the most cost-effective approaches (for example, family stress management plus pharmacotherapy for clients with schizophrenia). Clients who did not respond to this kind of early intervention were helped by extensive care at home. Falloon *et al.* (1987) indicated that this model of care proved a highly effective way of meeting the mental health needs of a community.

Table 9.2 *Some common 'lessons' or outcomes attributed to analytic psychotherapy*

1. **The world is not such a bad place after all**: people may be partly bad, but they are more reliable and trustworthy than had previously been experienced.

2. **To demand is to be unhappy**: others resent and react negatively to exploitation; it is necessary to reduce demands and accept limitations in oneself and others.

3. **It's not that bad**: suffering, anxiety, depression, etc. are not as bad as one had thought. Clients learn to credit themselves for their strength and endurance, and to face up to their problems.

4. **Honesty is a good policy**: openness about one's feelings and motives, no matter how unpleasant or 'immoral', helps with their acceptance and the choice of appropriate action.

5. **Accept authority**: one needs to accept and respect those in higher positions. It is futile to aggress, compete with or rebel against them. Better to accept their authority so freeing one from fruitless struggles.

6. **Accept responsibility**: it is self-defeating and ineffectual to blame others for one's predicament. One's social worth depends on what one does, and accepting responsibility permits one to take appropriate steps.

Effort evaluation

As the name suggests, this is concerned with the activities, resources and energy invested in a service. Thus, an effort evaluation of an individual care plan might indicate how many nurses spent how much time in various different ways on the care plan. To illustrate, Marks (1985) provided some effort data in his study of psychiatric nurse therapists in primary care. In the case of a client with an eating phobia, the nurse provided nine therapy sessions totalling 10 hours of therapist time.

The same kind of information can be provided for wards, units or services as a whole. For instance, a day hospital in which I worked had a programme of 13 activities, including handicrafts, relaxation training, dance therapy and a social skills group. An effort evaluation of this unit would detail these activities, who conducted them and for how long, thus allowing the evaluation to estimate the cost of the programme per client. It also allows the evaluator to estimate what this effort yields in terms of other types of evaluation, such as outcome or acceptability. Thus, one might compare the current programme on a ward with a revised one, in terms of its acceptability to the clients. To illustrate, I compared the psychiatric day hospital just mentioned with a second one in another district in terms of programmes, clients and outcomes (Milne, 1984). One of the units had far fewer clients and activities, though both were similar at the levels of client functioning. When re-assessed three months later, the more active day hospital appeared to have produced better results with its clients. As both units had similar staffing levels and resources, it seemed that the better results were due to a more varied and active programme in one of the day hospitals. This example indicates how evaluations of effort (number and types of activities, staff and clients) can usefully relate to evaluations of outcome.

Effort data are therefore relatively easy to gather. However, care should be taken in their interpretation, as it does not necessarily follow that more effort always yields better results. An analogy which I find helpful is that of a car wheel which is stuck in the mud. Although the wheel may spin at great speed, the car stays put: the effort or work which is being done achieves nothing, and may even make matters worse. For this reason, effort data are probably the least useful of all five forms of evaluation when conducted in isolation. They are at their best when combined with others, since this greatly helps with the interpretation of outcome or efficiency evaluations.

Process evaluation

Traditionally, a focus on therapeutic *process* has dominated the literature of evaluation, providing highly detailed accounts of what takes place during therapy. However, these accounts have tended to be descriptive rather than evaluative, as relatively little attention is paid to goals or outcomes.

Although there have been more combined process and outcome evaluations latterly, there is still a tendency for researchers to focus on one at the expense of the other. This focus is usually on outcome. Thus, it is common to find articles which describe the outcomes achieved by a particular programme, without specifying how this was achieved. In one review of journal articles it was found that the majority did not involve any check on whether or not the intervention actually corresponded to its label, while a sizeable minority did not even define the intervention beyond a general label, such as 'cognitive therapy' (Peterson *et al.*, 1982). In practice, there is scope for large differences in the interpretation of these terms. To illustrate, Salkovskis (1987) reported that one study had claimed to employ cognitive therapy, but that in effect this consisted of an intervention lasting between one and two minutes!

In my own experience, careful analysis of my therapy process revealed that I was practising behavioural rather than the cognitive-behavioural therapy I had believed I was employing (Milne, 1989).

The process evaluation model I had applied in that study indicated that the *skill*, *type* and *interpersonal effectiveness* of the therapist were the most important variables to assess (Schaffer, 1982). *Skill* refers to the level of competence; *type* to the goals and tactics of a therapy; while *interpersonal effectiveness* covers the quality of the therapist–client relationship. Different instruments can be used to measure each of these variables. In the example of my study I used the *Cognitive Therapy Scale* (Young and Beck, 1980) to measure the skill dimension, the *Helper Behaviour Rating Scale* (Hardy and Shapiro, 1985; see also Chapter 6) to define the type of therapy, and a consumer satisfaction questionnaire which in part gauged interpersonal effectiveness. The relevant satisfaction items are set out in *Table 9.3*.

Process evaluations can also focus on units or whole services, in each case considering the basic question: What goes on here? This goes beyond the effort evaluation's focus on the *content* of a care plan (the methods, such as 'cognitive therapy', used to promote change) to consider how this is conducted. But as the example shows, effort and process can overlap, as seen when asking what type of therapy is being provided.

As an illustration of a process evaluation at the systems level, consider the study reported by Sanson-Fisher and Jenkins (1978) and previously mentioned in Chapter 7. They observed the interactions between staff and clients in a penal institution for delinquent girls in Australia. It appeared that although the unit's programme dictated that the girls should be occupied in 'therapeutic opportunities' (such as household chores), in practice the girls coerced the staff into doing the chores for them! For instance, the staff spent 88 per cent of their time 'passively watching' and 'talking positively' to the girls when they were *not* doing the chores, while the girls gave positive attention to the staff when they did the chores 97 per cent of the time. When the staff tried to reverse the position towards the unit's objectives they faced 'aversive' control by the girls (swearing and physical threats).

Process evaluation of this kind helps us to understand the relationship between effort and outcome, the way in which different amounts of

Table 9.3 *Items from a consumer satisfaction questionnaire used to measure the 'interpersonal effectiveness' of a therapist*

Item

- I found it easy to understand the psychologist
- Other people would approve of the way the psychologist worked
- Appointments should be shorter
- The appointments were conducted in a satisfactory manner

---

resources (for example, time, staffing levels, and expertise) relate to various outcomes. In this example, Sanson-Fisher and Jenkins (1978) were able to define what they observed as a coercion process, which explained why the unit was not achieving expected outcomes. This led naturally to recommendations, including specialised training for the staff in such areas as discriminating between appropriate and inappropriate client behaviour; in developing their ability to control their reactions; and in obtaining the necessary support for such changes from their own supervisors.

Efficiency evaluation

No matter how well a care plan or a service works, there is almost always scope for improvement. This might take the form of less effort (fewer days as an in-patient) or a different process (the use of self-help materials) in order to achieve the same outcome. Or it may be possible to improve matters by increasing effort in order to achieve an even better result.

I realise that, at the time of writing, the term 'efficiency' is steeped in political connotations, as it is often used as a euphemism for closing down wards and cutting back on services. (The same applies to the term 'cost improvement'.) This is an unfortunate exploitation of the term, for efficiency is a wholesome objective in all walks of life, and most mental health professionals will have a natural concern to promote it. They will be interested in learning how to make their service go further, and how to make it work more smoothly and more effectively, because they believe in what they do and they recognise the great unmet need of the community in which they work.

As discussed earlier, services such as the Buckinghamshire one (Falloon *et al.*, 1987) are clearly concerned with efficiency. The project team want to know how their home-based approach compares to the traditional hospital-based one, in terms of its outcomes and efficiency. Their overriding concern is to do a better job in providing more effective care. They are justified in assuming that such an improvement is possible, given the plentiful illustrations of this in the past. In general medicine, for example, special coronary care units were found to be no better than much less expensive home-based care (Mather *et al.*, 1971). In community psychiatric nursing, Mangen *et al.* (1983) found evidence to indicate that the CPN service was less expensive than out-patient psychiatric appointments, with no difference in clinical outcome. They considered chronic 'neurotic' clients during a follow-up phase and took account of such costs as the use of the general practitioner, of day centres, unemployment and sickness benefits, travel costs, and so forth. As well as being cheaper, the CPN service was more highly regarded by the clients.

A weakness of this kind of evaluation is that one immediately wants to ask about the respective services, in order to consider the appropriateness of the comparison. This is a process question, and so it again underlines the importance of combining a process evaluation with outcome or efficiency evaluations. Efficiency is therefore an important but inconclusive aspect of service evaluation.

Acceptability evaluation

Measurement of client satisfaction or the acceptability of a service is also problematic, though important. The fundamental difficulty is that clients invariably make very positive ratings, seemingly regardless of the service concerned. This has been attributed to a pressure on them to provide a 'grateful testimonial' for a service that is free at the point of access (such as the NHS). Other factors are the absence of any plausible comparison points: unlike other services, such as those provided by garages or hotels, the client is unlikely to have sampled a range of mental health sevices. Related to this is the kind of limited expectations the client might be expected to have about the effectiveness of such a service in any case (that is, they are not generally reputed to offer a rapid 'cure'). Other considerations include a client's wish not to repay the kindness and care they have received by criticism. For such reasons, evaluations of a services acceptability have earned a cautious interpretation.

A sobering illustration of the potential for acceptability data to mislead has been provided by Parker and Thomas (1980). They found that those students who learned the most, rated their instructors least favourably, while conversely those who learned the least gave the highest ratings! Similarly, Lebow's (1982) review included reports of wide variations between client and therapist ratings of clinical outcomes.

However, some of these difficulties can be minimised, as discussed by Lebow (1982). One suggestion is to state on the form that the service providers will not be adversely affected by the client's ratings. Another is to make it clear that only the average rating provided will be fed back to the providers by a third party, thus freeing the client to offer a more candid opinion. A third option is to seek information on a range of aspects of a service, and not just focus on general, overall satisfaction. Although some dispute remains in the evaluation literature as to whether 'acceptability' is a uni- or a multidimensional concept, there is an emerging consensus that, for practical purposes at least, a form with multiple dimensions is more useful. Examples include the process, content, outcome, and goals of a service, and the speed with which it is provided, together with the competence of the staff (Nguyen *et al.*, 1983). By introducing such multidimensionality, clients are provided with plausible comparison points (for example, a client could express high satisfaction with the process and content, but regard the outcome as less acceptable). When considering the results, staff are also able to relate one set of scores to another. Finally, to take account of the Parker and Thomas (1980) finding, acceptability ratings should be considered alongside 'harder' data, such as learning or symptomatic improvement (that is, outcome data).

Turning from the problematic nature of acceptability evaluation to the question of its importance, there appears to be unanimity amongst service providers and users that it is a necessary element of evaluation. This is firstly because an unacceptable service will deter clients, making subsequent issues like effort and outcome irrelevant. Other reasons include the fact that the client provides a unique perception of a service, one intrinsically relevant to service providers; and 'consumerism': the onus in judging services has shifted increasingly towards the client (as exemplified in the UK by the recent policy statements such as the White Paper *Caring for People*).

On balance, then, a service evaluation should include an acceptability assessment, probably best set out in a multidimensional format and related to at least an outcome evaluation, in order to facilitate interpretation of the results.

The steps in evaluation

Earlier I defined evaluation in terms of a number of steps, foremost amongst which was the identification of the goals of a care plan or service. I now propose to take a closer look at these steps, alongside some of the more common difficulties that arise and some of the possible solutions. The points are equally applicable to direct work with individuals or services, and I will give examples of both. Each step draws on a particular type of evaluation, as set out above.

Identifying goals

Given the definition of evaluation in terms of the extent to which goals are achieved, it would appear rather obvious that goal specification is crucial. Yet many people attempt to evaluate when no such clarity exists, while others may lose sight of clear goals during the evaluation process. If you think back to the different types of evaluation and the questions they address (for example 'Did the care plan work?'; 'How much effort did it take to achieve the objective?'), they can all be seen as relative to the original aim of the intervention. Clinicians can be forgiven their inconsistency over goal setting, as good examples from managers within their organisations are not often forthcoming. More commonly, managers simply offer bland 'philosophies of care', such as 'helping individuals to achieve the highest possible level of independence'. These philosophies can be useful if they identify the broad values and aims of a service or unit, but they need to be translated into specific 'performance' statements to serve an evaluation role (see Chapter 3 for a reminder of 'fuzzies' and 'performances'). The aim is to reduce ambiguity as far as possible, while pinpointing appropriate objectives. These objectives should be set out in a way that allows one to check whether or not progress is being made, and ultimately whether the objectives are attained. Stating objectives clearly can also help others to work towards them. It is against these criteria that statements such as 'the highest possible level of independence' fall short.

Other criteria have been listed by Ward (1985). These include the need to have objectives which are client-centred, easily attainable, provable, quantitative and time-limited. As illustrations, he provides several case studies. These include such objectives as:

- 'will sleep for three, two-hourly periods per 24 hours'
- 'can remember the name of the interviewing nurse'
- 'will hold a one-minute conversation with each shift nurse per half day'
- 'will review a daily newspaper with nursing staff'

As these examples indicate, the principles of goal setting apply equally to individuals or services.

Exercise 9.2: Assessing goals in care plans
As an exercise, list and define the criteria for goal setting examined in this section before applying them to a random sample of care plans. When you find poor examples try to note a more adequate alternative.

Analysing service tasks

Having defined a care plan or service goal, the next step in evaluation is to consider how best to achieve it. This mirrors the planning stage of the nursing process, particularly in the analysis of a problem, as stressed in Chapter 5. A classic example from work in institutions is the question of whether a client's 'challenging behaviour' is the 'problem', or whether the behaviour is identifying a problem in the way the client is being treated. In both cases, the objective might be to eliminate the challenging behaviour, but the task is quite different depending on the analysis. Similarly, in resettling long-stay clients one might be faced with opposition from the neighbours of a community home. Is the problem the 'odd appearance' that they point to in the clients, or the neighbours' attitudes to the mentally ill? Either way, the goal is to successfully settle the clients in their new abode.

A generally less exacting task than analysing a service is that of describing the client group. Indeed, this should be regarded as the first stage of the analysis. What kinds of difficulties are the clients experiencing? Which types of needs are paramount? How many of them fall into each category? By breaking down the clients in this way one can gain an overview of the task facing a ward or a service. Although relatively straightforward, this description can highlight some surprising discrepancies between what is needed and what is provided. To illustrate, a summary of the referral information on over 70 day hospital clients revealed that anxiety was the most commonly identified difficulty, yet little was provided to deal with it (Milne, 1987). (This step is similar to 'needs assessment' discussed in Chapter 3.)

Describing and standardising services

Just as it can prove helpful to describe the client group, so evaluation is aided by descriptions of the intervention. To know that 70 per cent of clients benefit from a service or a particular kind of care plan begs the question of what was done in order to achieve this impressive result. It is necessary, therefore to obtain clear and objective specifications of the work done. For example, 'reality orientation', 'counselling', 'anxiety management' and 'cognitive therapy' are all somewhat vague terms for describing an intervention. They serve adequately as brief forms of communication, but are inadequate as an account of a care plan as a unit's programme: it is relatively easy to think of the different forms that these interventions can take. The problem lies partly in measuring the amount of work done, as exemplified by effort evaluation.

In addition to measuring what was done, sound evaluation requires *standardisation*, that is, the consistent application of an assessment or therapy. This is not so pronounced in individual care plans, although even at this level different nurses may implement a given plan or model in different ways. At the level of a ward or service these challenges can become even more significant as, for example, different disciplines interpret their role in discrepant ways. Another common factor over the longer time periods considered in evaluation is staff changes. This may alter not only what is done but also the way in which it is done (take, for example, the enthusiasm generated by a new colleague).

As before, it is often easier to try to describe the service than to regulate it. Provided a good record is maintained of what was done, it is often possible retrospectively to tease out the key features and relate these to outcomes. Indeed, the unplanned changes to a programme of

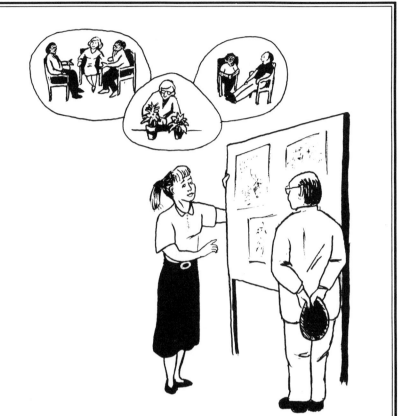

It is useful to describe a service as clearly as possible

care may function as natural experiments, indicating better ways of working. The overriding aim is to monitor what is done in a way which will at least allow one to say whether it did or did not correspond to a 'standard'. (Chapter 6 contained a detailed example, using the *Helper Behaviour Rating System* to describe what the therapist did.)

Measuring the amount of change that occurs

There are many ways of measuring the thoughts, feelings and behaviours of clients, although much remains to be done to improve instruments. Chapter 4 contained a summary of the main assessment methods, such as interviewing and observing. Many of these can also serve as evaluation tools, in the sense that they may be administered at the beginning and end of a care plan. The initial administration can serve to define difficulties and objectives, while the later one measures the amount of change that has occurred. To return to the example from psychiatric rehabilitation provided by Stanley (1984), reassessment of a client by means of the goal attainment scale allows the nurse to evaluate the client's progress at different stages during the implement-ation of the care plan.

Other potentially suitable instruments are presented in scientific journals and in text books or manuals (see the Further Reading list). *Table 9.4* lists a range of measures relevant to mental health nursing.

A more difficult task than obtaining a suitable evaluation instrument

Table 9.4 *Some readily available clinical measures*

Type of measure	Examples	What it measures	Source
Questionnaire	Mobility inventory for agoraphobia	Agoraphobic avoid-ance and frequency of panic attacks	Chambless *et al.* (1985)
	Depression inventory	Depression	Beck *et al.* (1961)
	Coping responses questionnaire	Cognitive, behavioural and affective ways of coping	Billings and Moos (1961)
	Self-efficacy scale	General and social effectiveness	Sherer *et al.* (1982)
	Dyadic adjustment scale	Quality of marriage and similar dyads	Spanier (1976)
Structured Interview	Social behaviour assessment schedule	Burden on relatives	Platt *et al.* (1980)
	Present state examination	Measurement and classification of psychiatric symptoms	Wing *et al.* (1970)
	Symptom rating scale	Rating of four aspects of chronic schizophrenia	Wing (1961)
Observation	Inpatient scale of minimal functioning	Low-level behaviour amongst chronic populations	Paul *et al.* (1976)
	Nurses' Observation Scale for Inpatient Evaluation	Higher levels of functioning amongst chronic population	Honigfeld (1966)

is its administration, in two senses. Firstly there can be problems associated with the demands of using the tool, as it may require special training or may be in some sense impractical (perhaps taking an hour per client to complete). Secondly there is a problem in that each evaluator administers a somewhat different set of instruments. This reflects the immature stage of development of the evaluation field, but has the drawback of making it difficult to compare results across services or settings. Some progress has been made with regard to certain problems, as in the wide acceptance of the *Beck Depression Inventory* (Beck *et al.*, 1961) as the common instrument for assessing depression. However, this kind of common practice is, unfortunately, the exception rather than the rule.

A simple alternative to the use of published measures is some form of direct observation record. This can be tailored towards each individual client, and consist of a note of the frequency, intensity, or duration of a specific behaviour, such as how long a compulsive washing ritual lasts, or how many times per hour a client asks for a cigarette. (I will return to this shortly, in discussing some case study research designs.) Measures of the kind outlined here, whether of the published or home-made (*ad hoc*) variety, are related to outcome evaluation, as described earlier.

Determining the extent to which change is due to the care plan

This refers to the isolation of the intervention from other kinds of help or influence which may be present. The concern is to clarify whether a '70 per cent improvement' is due to the care plan or to other changes. It is of course tempting to assume that the work one does as a nurse is the most powerful factor when a client improves. However, the effects of medication, social support and, in diverse ways, 'the passage of time' may sometimes be more powerful. In one sobering survey, Freeman and Button (1984) found evidence of a 'worst year' phenomenon: clients presenting with psychological problems to their GP tended to be 'better' a year later, even when there was no significant intervention. In short, there appears to be a natural process of crisis and resolution for some primary care difficulties. Those who evaluate the effectiveness of their work in this context, therefore, need to take account of this kind of phenomenon.

Given that evaluation typically affords far less control over the key elements of a study than does laboratory research, it is not surprising that evaluators have difficulty deciding on cause and effect in their work. These key elements of cause and effect are more properly referred to in science as the *independent* and *dependent* variables, respectively. The independent variable is the one that is manipulated or which is regarded as the intervention, while the dependent variable is the measure or impact of this intervention. I have already touched on some of the difficulties in controlling the independent variable in the section on standardising programmes (and in Chapter 6), not to mention the other variables which can cause change in the client at the same time as the care plan (for example, the effects of medication or social support). I also indicated that dependent variables were not without their drawbacks, although the use of simple observational data affords a practical yet systematic approach. Allied to comparably straightforward research designs, such data can allow one to judge the cause and effect of a care plan or service.

Before considering case study research designs, let me mention one other practical way of judging the impact of your care plan. This entails measuring the specific variable that you expect to influence through your care plan. That is, in contrast to a general measure, such as the *Beck Depression Inventory*, one targets a more discrete factor for both the evaluation and the care plan. For instance, if the problem is depression, a cognitive therapy approach might be seen as appropriate. This being so, one might measure the kinds of dysfunctional thoughts believed to cause and maintain the depression. Similarly, instead of measuring the broad variable 'anxiety', one might focus on panic attack frequency. *Table 9.4* contains examples of such instruments.

The logic underlying the use of specific measures is that while social support, changes in medication and so on will probably influence such general conditions as anxiety or depression, they are unlikely to impinge directly on the specific focus of a care plan. An example is to follow the stress–coping–strain model set out in Chapter 1. This allows one to record changes in stressors while noting the impact of the intervention on a client's coping strategies. If successful in improving coping, there should be a resultant improvement in 'strain' (that is, distress).

However, the main option for increasing your confidence that a care plan or nursing service has produced a change is to apply your measures within a *research design*. This is a strategy which reduces the risk that factors other than the one you are interested in (the independent variable) are responsible for the results you observe (the dependent variable). A consideration of research design therefore belongs in this section, but because it is a large topic I have deferred it to the end of the section (p222) in order to maintain the present emphasis on the steps in evaluation.

Assessing the relative effectiveness of modified programmes

The ultimate stage in Suchman's (1967) breakdown of evaluative research looks at the success of various forms of a service. This may follow from having established that a care plan is producing the desired effect (for example '70 per cent improvement' in a client's orientation) and wanting to find out whether there is a better way of achieving this sort of result. Alternatively, two new forms of intervention might be compared. This is therefore closest to efficiency evaluation, as described earlier in this chapter.

The best way to find out if there is 'a better way' is by comparing two or more care plans in relation to similar clients. This is not as simple as it sounds, since it can prove difficult to equalise the care plans or the clients on all the important variables. Consequently, it is not surprising to find that there are few published attempts at comparing two programmes of care (*comparative evaluations*).

One of the rare examples has been provided by Brooker and Simmons (1985), who compared two CPN teams working in Bloomsbury Health Authority. One team was based at a day hospital, while the second worked from health centres and clinics. The researchers compared the types of clients and caseload activities of these two teams, finding differences in both variables. Social isolation and deprivation were higher amongst the clients of the day hospital based CPNs, indicating some important differences between the two groups of clients. Also, this team of CPNs spent significantly less time in clinical contact with their clients, in particular with regard to home visits.

Brooker and Simmons noted that such differences have been found to affect the level of client satisfaction. In this sense, then, the 'modified' (non-traditional, health-centre based) programme of community psychiatric nursing can be seen to deal with different clients in a somewhat different way. It appears to be more effective in providing community-based care (home visits), and so the service's managers might decide to emphasise it more in the future. As the authors stress, this is a good example of how evaluation can help to shape policy and practice.

Collaboration in evaluation

Before leaving this section I would like to emphasise briefly an important step in evaluation which is implicit in the preceding discussion. This concerns the role of other people – collaborators – in service evaluation. It is often the case that evaluations are done 'to' services or 'on' nurses by outside experts. In contrast, I have placed the onus on the individual nurse as the evaluator, whether of a care plan or a larger service unit, such as a CPN team. This emphasis is consistent with the philosophy of the 'knowledgeable doer' as the product of Project 2000. It carries with it the important implication that the evaluation is directly relevant to clinical practice and will stand a far better chance of improving practice than will the findings provided by outside experts.

This is not to say that there is no place for collaborators in evaluation. Obviously some professions tend to have more research experience than others (for example, clinical psychologists). The issue is therefore how best to harness such resources. One promising approach is called *stakeholder-collaborative evaluation* (Ayers, 1987). This consists of an extended role for service providers (the 'stakeholders') in evaluation, including designing, implementing and interpreting the research aided by an external evaluator (the 'collaborator'). This kind of teamwork may be facilitating for nurses during any of Suchman's six steps in evaluation.

Research designs

Mention has already been made of research designs, as for example in helping us to determine the extent to which a care plan produces improvements in the client. Is it just the healing passage of time, or the gradual impact of medication that explains this improvement? How can we tease out cause and effect sufficiently to have some confidence in the effect of our work? In essence the answer lies in carefully designed evaluations. These are ones in which we can exclude the major alternatives to our intervention, such as chemotherapy, leaving us with more confidence that our work was indeed the reason for the observed improvement.

First I will summarise some *single-subject* ($N = 1$) research designs ('subject' is the traditional term for a person in an experiment, while 'N' refers to the sample size), and then I will go on to consider research designs for the evaluation of groups of clients and for indirect work.

Single-subject research designs

There are several major types of single-subject research designs, but they all share certain procedures (Hersen and Barlow, 1976), as summarised in *Table 9.5*. Before studying the Table, please note that 'A' refers to a *baseline* period, that is, time when a behaviour, thought or feeling is recorded at its natural, pre-intervention level. In contrast, 'B' refers to an intervention phase, such as putting up signs to help orientate a client. Any additional interventions, such as a reality-orientation programme, are given consecutive letters (C, D, and so on), although, as I will point out shortly, these are usually interspersed by a reversion to baseline (thus giving 'ABAC' designs). All single-subject designs represent an improvement on the traditional case study, which

Table 9.5 *Key procedures in single subject research designs*

Procedure	Description
1. Repeated measurement	Because changes do not tend to follow a smooth pattern it is necessary to measure repeatedly over time.
2. Choosing a baseline	During this repeated measurement one typically starts with a baseline phase. This provides a standard against which the impact of an intervention can be contrasted.
3. Changing one variable at a time	A baseline is maintained until the variable/s of interest become stable or predictable. Then one intervention is introduced at a time so as to avoid confounding the effects of two or more interventions.
4. Reversal and withdrawal	Once an intervention has been introduced it can be removed, so reverting to baseline (an ABA design or withdrawal); or it can be reinstated (ABAB or reversal design).
5. Phase length	Baseline and intervention phases of measurement should be maintained until there is some stability to the data. This allows clear conclusions to be drawn about the effect of the intervention.

is an intervention (that is, 'B' phase) without the benefit of a proper baseline.

Multiple phase designs

From these basic procedures it is possible to construct a range of research designs, classed as *multiple phase* designs. The simplest is an AB design, in which a baseline (A) is taken prior to an intervention (B). However, this is a weak design as it is quite possible that a third variable (C) has had an impact on the client at the same time as the intervention that you have introduced. In order to overcome this difficulty, a withdrawal design can be used, 'ABA'. If the data follow the kind of pattern illustrated in *Figure 9.1*, then one has more confidence that the intervention was indeed responsible for the observed effect.

However, a withdrawal design is basically impractical, as one typically wants to stop the evaluation at a point when clients are in a phase where they are benefiting from the care plan. For this reason an 'ABAB' or *reversal* design is more appropriate. It is also more convincing or rigorous than the 'AB' or 'ABA' designs. Ideally a follow-up period is added after the final intervention phase, such as another assessment three or six months after the end of the intervention. This establishes whether the effects of the care plan have lasted, an important criterion by which to judge any intervention.

A popular variant of the 'ABAB' design is the 'ABCB' design. This allows one to compare the effectiveness of two interventions on the same client. For instance, an elderly confused client may respond fairly well to the orientation signs ('B' phase in *Figure 9.1*) but not

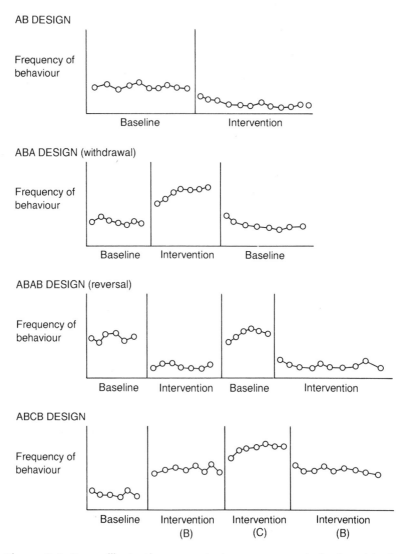

Figure 9.1 *Some illustrative, repeated measurement single subject designs, based on imaginary data on the frequency of a behaviour in relation to various interventions.*

sufficiently well to always find the toilet. The vertical axis in this example might therefore be a measure of the client's success in locating the toilet (frequency of successful trips). One could then try a different approach, such as verbal prompting (intervention 'C'), and, if successful, this would yield a picture such as that in the 'ABCB' design in *Figure 9.1*. Hersen and Barlow (1976) provide many variations on these multiple phase designs, together with illustrative material drawn from the research literature.

Multiple baseline designs

Hersen and Barlow (1976) also provide examples from a different class of single-subject designs, called *multiple baseline designs*. These maintain the procedures listed in *Table 9.5*, such as repeated measurement, but they differ by measuring more than one thing at a time. This can be different behaviours, different clients, or the same client in different settings. For these reasons they are referred to as *multiple baseline across behaviours* and so forth. To continue the example of the preceding paragraph, an illustration of this design would be to evaluate changes in the elderly confused person's ability to locate the toilet, alongside the person's ability to wash and feed themselves. In contrast, a *multiple baseline across clients* might compare a group of matched elderly people in terms of their response to an intervention; while a *multiple baseline across settings* might consider whether a client's improvements in orientation in the ward were also obtained in other parts of the hospital.

All of these multiple baseline designs share an advantage over repeated measures approaches in that they do not require a withdrawal or reversal phase in order to provide a convincing demonstration of cause and effect. This demonstration comes from effectively treating those things which are not being addressed as 'controls'. Thus, in the example of the elderly confused client, the other self-help behaviours of the client, the response of other clients, or the client's own response to different settings would each provide evidence on the effect of an intervention. If there were a confounding or third variable present (for example, the presence of some new clients), it would be unlikely to affect these recorded variables in quite the same way as the intervention. For example, the arrival of new clients would either have no impact on the client's orientation, or a general influence (say if a new client made a point of helping out). Either eventuality would have a rather different effect on the multiple baseline than would a nursing intervention.

The crucial reason for this is that in multiple baseline designs one alters only one variable at a time, for example focusing on one client until a steady result has been obtained before intervening with the

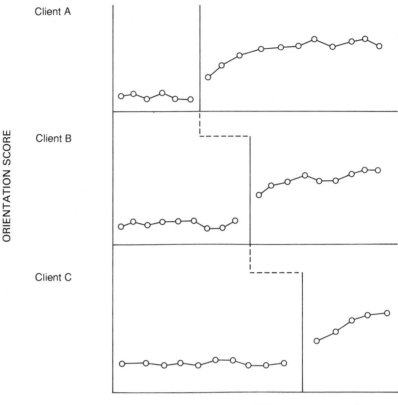

Figure 9.2 *An illustration of a 'multiple baseline across clients' research design. The imaginary intervention has been introduced first with Client A, then B, then C.*

second and third client. *Figure 9.2* shows how such a multiple baseline across behaviours might look for this example.

Exercise 9.3: Charting a care plan evaluation
A nurse's care plan evaluation took the form of a multiple phase research design. During the baseline phase, the client's personal hygiene ratings were: 2, 4, 3, 2, 3, 3, 2, 2, 4, 2. The nurse then introduced a programme of prompting the client to wash and shave, which yielded the following daily ratings: 4, 6, 7, 6, 8, 9, 8, 9, 7, 9. A reversal phase then resulted in a return to baseline rating: 4, 3, 2, 3, 2, 3, 3, 3, 4, 2. This convinced the nurse that the prompting programme was effective, and it was reinstated to produce this final series of ratings: 5, 7, 9, 8, 9, 10, 9, 9, 9, 9. Try to set these ratings out in a chart, as in *Figure 9.1*. How might you set

out the results from a supplementary care plan, in which the nurse moves on to tackle the client's social skills and recreational skills? That is, what kind of research design would be appropriate, and which sort of data could be gathered?

Group research designs

There are a large number of possible research designs, but these can be broken down into quasi-experimental and true experimental designs. In drawing this distinction, Campbell and Stanley (1963) suggested that the random allocation of clients or therapists to different interventions was the essential difference between the two types of design.

In this sense, some single-subject research designs are experimental, whereas others are only quasi-experimental. As you would expect, it is the designs which have most control built in that are classed as experimental. These include the multiple baseline and multiple phase designs. In contrast, the 'AB' single subject design is regarded as quasi-experimental because it has little control. To put this another way, in an 'AB' design it is hard to rule out a variety of other explanations for changes that might be observed during phase 'B'.

A study by Brooker and Simmons (1985) illustrates the quasi-experimental category for two groups, as the two teams of CPNs that they studied were not randomly allocated to either their day hospital or health centre bases. Had they been, one would have had more confidence that it was not something to do with the CPNs themselves that led them to be members of one team rather than another. For example, one might speculate that the CPNs who worked from a day hospital base were less interested in community care and so carried out fewer home visits. This motivational factor, rather than the base, may conceivably have explained the results. In contrast, Lavender's (1987) study (discussed in the next section) was based on randomisation and therefore fell into the experimental design category.

Factors to be controlled

Although there are a large number of variables, such as motivation, which can be the main effect in a study, in practice a limited number of factors tend to be considered. If one can control for the effect of these, or rule them out in other ways, then one can infer that the intervention did indeed cause the observed effect. This issue is referred to as *internal validity*, the extent to which one can attribute an effect to a known cause. It is strongest when all the alternative causes are controlled for, and weakest when there are many that are uncontrolled.

When a research design is weak, it is difficult to interpret the results with any confidence.

To illustrate, the *randomised controlled trial*, used most commonly in evaluating drugs, has the strongest internal validity as its design systematically excludes all the alternative causes. An 'AB' design (or pre-test and post-test only group research design), by comparison, has the weakest internal validity as it controls for none of these alternatives. Campbell and Stanley's (1963) famous text sets out the seven main factors that should be controlled in an evaluation. These are presented in *Table 9.6*.

They then related these to threats to the external validity of a study, namely factors which limit the extent to which the results apply to other situations (for example, to different clients or hospitals). External

Table 9.6 *Campbell and Stanley's (1963) list of factors to be controlled in an evaluation*

Factor	Definition
1. History	Any event occurring between assessment points, excluding the intervention.
2. Maturation	The effect of the passage of time on those being studied (for example growing older and wiser).
3. Testing	One consequence of an initial assessment is that people respond to it differently next time. For example, it makes them look things up in books or ask others about the assessment.
4. Instrumentation	Another measurement problem is that the instrument or measurement procedure may change between assessments, causing false readings (e.g. observers or raters who become more generous or careless with each assessment).
5. Statistical regression	When two groups are selected because of their extreme scores (for example 'depressed' versus 'normals') then there is a tendency for both groups of scores to revert to more average scores over time.
6. Selection	Comparison groups selected in a different way from the experimental group introduces a selection bias.
7. Experimental mortality	For reasons such as the differential selection of people for groups, they may be lost at different rates by the time of a re-assessment.

validity therefore concerns the generality or representativeness of a finding. To illustrate, if the clients who enter a therapy trial are atypical of those who are seen routinely in psychiatric out-patient departments, then one questions whether the marvellous results of the trial are not due to these 'special' clients. Many researchers do select their clients, making this a common issue. For example, Marks' (1985) evaluation of nurse therapists in primary care applied seven client selection criteria, which reduced the 254 referred clients to 150. The criteria included whether the client was likely to respond to therapy, and the absence of severe depression. Anyone studying these findings is bound to ask whether the 150 clients on whom they were based were representative of those seen routinely by nurse therapists in public services such as the NHS. To the extent that they are not representative, the study has low external validity: it proves something in relation to one time and place, but the results would probably not be replicated in another.

Campbell and Stanley (1963) related these threats systematically to the internal and external validity of a range of research designs. This indicated the strengths and weaknesses of each design. A few common designs will now be used to illustrate their systematic approach.

Common research designs

'Before and after' evaluation of one group

This is a widely used design, similar to the single subject 'AB' design. It suffers the same weaknesses in internal validity, such as the possibility that some third factor has produced any change between the two assessment points. For this reason it is not classed as a true experimental design, although it is better than a post-test evaluation alone.

'Before and after' control group design

By adding a second group to the preceding design one succeeds in controlling for all the threats to the internal validity of a study. This makes it a true experimental design. Clients should be allocated randomly to either the treated group or the control group. Both groups are assessed at the same time points, before and after the treatment.

'After assessment only' control group design

This only differs from the preceding design in omitting the initial pre-testing (or baseline). It is equally high in internal validity, but stronger in external validity as the assessment instruments have only been administered once. This prevents the clients from reacting in some way to the initial assessment thus influencing the post-testing.

As well as reducing the impact of assessment, this post-test only design is often more practical, and can be used when pre-tests are considered inappropriate (as when something quite new is being introduced).

Multiple time series

In this last example, the assessments are repeated at regular intervals before and after the intervention for an experimental and a control group. This does not require the random allocation of clients to groups, as repeated testing (at least three assessments before and after the treatment) will reveal their relative positions, enabling one to infer with considerable confidence whether there has been a treatment effect.

A case study

I discussed the evaluation of direct work with a ward manager catering for the less dependent psychiatric rehabilitation client, providing short-term accommodation and care for up to 18 clients with a diagnosis of schizophrenia or manic depression. Individual care plans are applied through a key worker system, including social skills training, counselling and family therapy. The ward has access to five homes to which the clients can move for the final phase of rehabilitation resettlement, as well as for providing respite care.

Outcome evaluation

The manager and his colleagues have developed an outcome evaluation system, based on the *Morningside Rehabilitation Status Scales* (Affleck and McGuire, 1984). Through careful consideration of the scales, first amongst the nursing staff and then through the multidisciplinary team, small changes were made to adapt them to the ward and its clients. The scales they ended up with are summarised in *Table 9.7.*

The evaluation procedure on the ward is for new clients to be assessed over an initial six-week period, during which time goals are set for each client. These goals are also defined by the scales. So, for example, in the case of a client with deficits on the *living skills scale*, a key worker might devise a care plan to achieve levels 1–2 (that is, 'able to demonstrate skills in using a washing machine and to iron clothes safely and correctly'). The present level of functioning can also be summarised quickly by the code for a different level. This system allows the nurses to readily establish baselines and goals for

Table 9.7 *A summary of* The Morningside Rehabilitation Status Scales *(Affleck and McGuire, 1984), as adapted and used by the nurses on the case study*

Scales	Illustrative levels
1. Current symptoms	Observable negative symptoms e.g. apathy, with-drawal or delusions (level 4)
2. Motivation	Has visited and identified place of resettlement (level 0)
3. Social integration	Has several established friends, other than ward/hospital based (level 1)
4. Self-care	Requires frequent prompting to promote self-care skills (level 4)
5. Living skills	Is able to prepare and cook meals providing a balanced diet (level 0)
6. Activity	Actively participates but does not initiate activities, as a rule (level 3)
7. Community contact	Uses community facilities (for example shopping, transport) occasionally without escort (level 2)
8. Physical disability	Mild disability may cause some difficulty (for example climbing stairs without assistance) (level 2)

each client in relation to the overall aims of the unit. Following a care plan, it allows them to evaluate its outcome, making it a coherent and attractively straightforward approach. The nurses regard it as a great success.

Figure 9.3 provides an illustration of the evaluation system in relation to a client whose key worker played a significant role in adapting the scales. The client had worked as a labourer and had spent periods in prison for theft. While in prison he was diagnosed as suffering from paranoid schizophrenia. Following a spell at home, where he was cared for by his sister, he was admitted to hospital. *Figure 9.3* provides a summary of the initial assessment of this client, indicating that he was functioning at a low level generally. He was spending much of the day lying in bed, refusing to work, and ignoring prompts regarding his personal hygiene.

Subsequent assessments made at monthly intervals, showed steady progress in most areas. By the final assessment he still had room for improvement in making 'community contacts' and reducing his isolation. However, the prospects seemed good that he would cope with self-catering accommodation in a house in the

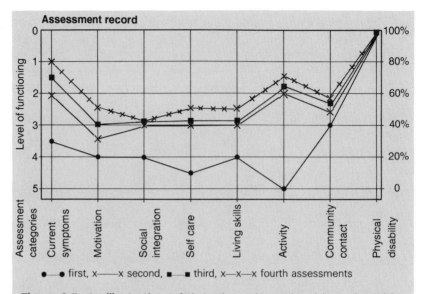

Figure 9.3 *An illustration of the adapted* Morningside Scale, *with assessments on a client at four time points.*

hospital grounds. If this was successful, he could move into a council flat in the community. In terms of research design, this represented an 'AB' single subject design.

Acceptability evaluation

As part of a management development course, the ward manager had also developed and applied a questionnaire measure of 'client satisfaction' on his ward. This was intended to analyse the quality of care that was provided. Only five areas of the ward's acceptability were assessed, as he did not want to make the questionnaire too stressful. The areas covered were: giving information to the client, the ward environment, catering, nursing staff and medical care.

The results, based on the replies of ten clients, indicated that the unit's acceptability was variable. Catering, for instance, was seen as poor (meals not very good, limited choice). More reassuringly, the nursing staff were rated very positively on their attitudes and work (being reassuring, informative and understanding). Interestingly, the questionnaire replies were more critical of the ward than were other sources of feedback (such as the residents meeting), which slightly surprised the staff and illustrated the value of different forms of evaluation. In general, however, the results indicated that the quality of care was acceptable to clients and in keeping with the unit's operational policy.

Some problems and solutions

As already touched upon, the ward manager went through a careful and gradual process of consultation with his nursing colleagues and the multidisciplinary team, noting and incorporating their comments into a revised set of scales. This made everyone in the team a 'stakeholder' and 'collaborator' in the new evaluation system, thereby increasing the likelihood of its successful implementation. This was enhanced by adapting the scales to suit the clients in the ward. Another common problem, that of incomplete care plan documentation, was reduced because of the ease and simplicity of recording goals, baselines and outcomes with the scales. There was also the added benefit of the scales making communication straightforward.

One problem the ward has yet to solve is how to obtain valid measures of a client's functioning in community settings, such as his or her own home. As the scales are applied in the relatively simple social context of a psychiatric hospital, it is not clear that the findings accurately reflect how a client functions in more complex environments, such as the High Street. A community rehabilitation team is being set up to address this sort of problem.

Summary

Evaluation concerns the systematic measurement of goal-attainment. Whether the goals are within an individual care plan or part of a large nursing service, the principles of evaluation can be applied. These include the different types of evaluation (for example, effort and outcome) and the steps to follow in evaluation (that is, starting with a measurable statement of the goal of an intervention). A key challenge in evaluation is research design, which provides the basis for judging whether an outcome is due to the intervention. The case study, drawn from a psychiatric rehabilitation ward, illustrates how nurses can adapt and successfully apply measures of outcome and acceptability within a 'before and after' research design.

Questions for further consideration

1 How would you define the goals of a nursing service such as a ward or community service?

2 Can you analyse the 'task' of a specific nursing service of your choice
   in such a way as to tease out a range of objectives, arranged in order
   of priority?
3 Taking the example of a client and care plan you know well, how
   might you measure changes in thoughts, feelings and behaviour?
4 What would a process–outcome evaluation of nursing care look
   like? Try to set out how you could measure both factors, based on a
   ward for elderly confused clients.
5 Some reasons were cited for the common finding that client
   satisfaction ratings tend to be favourable. Can you suggest which
   reasons you think best explain this phenomenon, and what you
   think can be done to obtain more accurate ratings?
6 Suggest suitable research designs for the following:
   a) Four long-stay clients who have similar levels of dependency and
      similar needs, and who are to move into a community hostel in
      pairs.
   b) Two groups of carers of clients with schizophrenia, one of which
      will represent a group receiving ten sessions of education and
      support.

References

Affleck, J. W. and McGuire, R. J. (1984). The measurement of psychiatric
   rehabilitation status: a review of the needs and a new scale. *British Journal of
   Psychiatry, 145*, 517–525.
Ayers, T. D. (1987). Stakeholders as partners in evaluation: a stakeholder–
   collaborative approach. *Evaluation and Program Planning, 10*, 263–271.
Barker, P. J. (1987). Evaluation in Nursing: the nurse as behaviour therapist.
   In D. L. Milne (Ed.) *Evaluating Mental Health Practice*. London:
   Croom Helm.
Barlow, D. H., Hayes, S. C. and Nelson, R. O. (1984). *The Scientist-Practitioner*.
   New York: Pergamon.
Beck, A. T., Ward, C. H., Mendelson, M., Mock, J. and Erbaugh, J. (1961). An
   inventory for measuring depression. *Archives of General Psychiatry, 4*,
   53–63.
Billings, A. G. and Moos, R. H. (1981). The role of coping responses and social
   resources in attenuating the stress of life events. *Journal of Behavioural
   Medicine, 4*, 139–157.
Brooker, C. and Simmons, S. (1985). A study to compare two models of
   community psychiatric nursing care delivery. *Journal of Advanced Nursing,
   10*, 217–223.
Campbell, D. T. and Stanley, J. C. (1963). *Experimental and quasi-experimental
   designs for research*. Chicago: Rand Mcnally.
Chambless, D. L., Caputo, G. C., Jasin, S. E., Gracely, E. J. and Williams, C.
   (1985). The mobility inventory for agoraphobia *Behaviour Research and
   Therapy, 23*, 35–44.
Falloon, I., Wilkinson, G., Burgess, J. and McLees, S. (1987). Evaluation in

Psychiatry: Planning, Developing and Evaluating Community-based Mental Health Services for Adults. In D. L. Milne (Ed.) *Evaluating Mental Health Practice*. London: Croom Helm.

Freeman, G. K. and Button, E. J. (1984). The clinical psychologist in general practice. *Journal of the Royal College of General Practitioners, 34,* 377–380.

Hardy, G. E. and Shapiro, D. A. (1985). Therapist response modes in prescriptive vs exploratory psychotherapy. *British Journal of Clinical Psychology, 24,* 235–245.

Hersen, M. and Barlow, D. H. (1976) *Single case experimental designs: strategies for studying behaviour change.* New York: Pergamon.

Honigfeld, G. (1966). *Nurses' Observation Scale for Inpatient Evaluation (NOSIE-30).* Glen Oaks, New York: Honigfeld.

Lavender, A. (1987). Improving the quality of care on psychiatric rehabilitation wards. *British Journal of Psychiatry, 150,* 476–481.

Lebow, J. (1982). Consumer satisfaction with mental health treament. *Psychological Bulletin, 91,* 244–259.

Luker, K. A. (1981). An overview of evaluation research in nursing. *Journal of Advanced Nursing, 6,* 87–93.

Mangen, S. P., Paykel, E. S., Griffith, J. H., Burchell, A. and Mancini, P. (1983). Cost-effectiveness of community psychiatric nurse or out-patient psychiatrist care of neurotic patients. *Psychological Medicine, 13,* 407–416.

Marks, I. M. (1985). *Psychiatric Nurse Therapists in primary care.* London: Royal College of Nursing.

Mather, H. G., Pearson, W. G., Read, K. L., Shaw, K. L. Q., Steed, D. B., Thorne, G. R., Jones, M. G., Guerrier, C. J., Eraut, C. D., McHugh, P. M., Chowdhury, N. R., Jafary, M. H. and Wallace, T. J. (1971). Acute myocardial infarction: home and hospital treatment. *British Medical Journal, 3,* 334.

Milne, D. L. (1984). A comparative evaluation of two psychiatric day hospitals *British Journal of Psychiatry, 145,* 533–537.

Milne, D. L. (1987). *Evaluating Mental Health Practice: Methods and Applications.* London: Croom Helm.

Milne, D. L. (1989). Multidimensional evaluation of therapist behaviour. *Behavioural Psychotherapy, 17,* 253–266.

Nguyen, T. D., Attkinson, C. C. and Stegner, B. L. (1983). Assessment of patient satisfaction: development and refinement of a service evaluation questionnaire. *Evaluation and Program Planning, 6,* 299–314.

Parker, R. M. and Thomas, K. R. (1980). Fads, flaws, fallacies and foolishness in evaluation of rehabilitation programmes. *Journal of Rehabilitation, 46,* 32–34.

Pattie, A. H. (1981). A survey version of the Clifton Assessment Procedures for the Elderly (CAPE). *British Journal of Clinical Psychology, 20,* 173–178.

Paul, E. L., Redfield, J. P. and Lentz, R. J. (1976). The inpatient scale of minimal functioning: a revision of the social breakdown syndrome gradient index. *Journal of Consulting and Clinical Psychology, 44,* 1021–1022.

Peterson, L., Homer, A. L. and Wonderlich, S. A. (1982). The integrity of independent variables in behaviour analysis. *Journal of Applied Behaviour Analysis, 15,* 477–492.

Platt, S., Weyman, A., Hirsch, S. and Hewett, S. (1980). The Social Behaviour Assessment Schedule (SBAS): rationale, contents, scoring and reliability, of a new interview schedule. *Social Psychiatry, 15,* 43–55.

Salkovskis, P. M. (1987). Cognitive therapy: is it always cognitive, is it always therapy? In H. R. Dent (Ed.) *Clinical Psychology: Research and Practice.* London: Croom Helm.

Sanson-Fisher, R. and Jenkins, H. J. (1978). Interaction patterns between inmates and staff in a maximum security institution for delinquents. *Behaviour Therapy, 9*, 703–716.

Schaffer, N. D. (1982). Multidimensional measures of therapist behaviour as predictors of outcome. *Psychological Bulletin, 92*, 670–681.

Sherer, M., Maddux, J. E., Mercandante, B., Prentice-Dunn, S., Jacobs, B. and Rogers, R. W. (1982). The self-efficacy scale: construction and validation *Psychological Reports, 51*, 663–671.

Spanier, G. B. (1976). Measuring dyadic adjustment: new scales for assessing the quality of marriage and similar dyads. *Journal of Marriage and the Family,* February, 15–27.

Stanley, B. (1984). Evaluation of treatment goals: the use of goal attainment scaling. *Journal of Advanced Nursing, 9*, 351–356.

Strupp, H. H. (1973). *Psychotherapy: clinical, research and theoretical issues.* New York: Jason Aronson.

Suchman, E. A. (1967). *Evaluative Research.* New York: Russell Sage.

Ward, M. F. (1985). *The Nursing Process in Psychiatry.* Edinburgh: Churchill Livingstone.

Wing, J. K. (1961). A simple and reliable subclassification of chronic schizophrenia. *Journal of Mental Science, 107*, 862–875.

Wing, J. K., Cooper, J. E. and Sartorius, N. (1974). *Measurement and Classification of Psychiatric Symptoms.* Cambridge: Cambridge University Press.

Young, J. E. and Beck, A. T. (1980). *Cognitive Therapy Scale.* Centre for Cognitive Therapy, University of Pennsylvania, Room 602, 133 South 36th Street, PA 19104, USA.

Further reading

Chenger, P. L. (1988). Collaborative nursing research – advantages and obstacles. *International Journal of Nursing Studies, 25*, 295–300.
This paper outlines the experience of collaboration between nurses in academic and clinical settings. Although Chenger identifies some benefits of this collaboration (such as enhancing the scientific base of nursing practice), she also notes some difficulties. These include the common problem of effective communication and the different objectives of the collaborators.

Lloyd, M. E. (1983). Selecting systems to measure client outcome in human service agencies. *Behaviour Assessment, 5*, 55–70.
Following Stanley's (1984) example, Lloyd considers five different kinds of instruments for measuring goal attainment. Amongst her criteria are sensitivity of the tool to client change and the utility of the information provided. She raises some fundamental questions about goal-attainment measures, such as the issue of goal-setting, in a stimulating and searching review.

Three books containing detailed descriptions and critiques of numerous measures are contained in the volumes below. In addition, they provide suggestions on the selection of appropriate instruments:

Goldstein, G. and Hersen, M. (1990). *Handbook of Psychological Assessment 2nd edn.* Windsor: NFER.

Hersen, M. and Bellack, A. A. (1988). *Dictionary of Behavioural Assessment Techniques.* Windsor: NFER.

Thompson, C. (Ed; 1989). *The Instruments of Psychiatric Research.* Chichester: Wiley.
This book offers a review of available measures including a summary and evaluation of a variety of measures of schizophrenia, anxiety and depression. Other major problem categories are also addressed in this way, as are more general issues of measurement, such as the design of rating scales and those surrounding the measurement of social and environmental determinants of mental health. This edited book is therefore a useful summary of measures and measurement issues, though it lacks examples of the instruments reviewed.

Milne, D. L. (1992). *Assessment: A Mental Health Portfolio.* Windsor: NFER.
This is a collection of questionnaires, rating scales and structured interviews ready for use in relation to the main problem categories in adult out-patient work (for example, anxiety, depression). It makes a set of sound and widely used measures readily available to clinicians, thus overcoming access and interpretation problems.

10 Evaluating indirect work

The main points made in the preceding chapter about the types of, and steps in, evaluation apply with equal strength to this chapter, while many of the points in this chapter also apply to Chapter 9. However, there are differences in the kind of measurement instrument used in indirect work and the work itself is also different. This chapter therefore considers examples of work in training, social support and institutional systems, and reviews a range of instruments and methods. In essence these raise the level of analysis from the individual to that of the group or system.

Why evaluate?

The most straightforward reply to this question has been given already: one evaluates in order to obtain systematic feedback, thus ensuring a rational basis for developing a care plan or a nursing service: it represents a form of professional learning. The alternative is to be guided by intuition or convention, neither of which sits comfortably with the principles of good practice, Project 2000 or general management.

This leads to a second motive for evaluation, namely that of the growing demand for 'accountable' services. Public attitudes, cutbacks in funding, the principles of 'good' nursing (for example, 'nursing standards') and 'good' management (for example, 'quality assurance' and 'control'), not to mention the increasing place of 'consumerism', have all raised the demand for accountability. Increasingly services have to be able to demonstrate that they are safe, appropriate and effective if they are to meet the standards of these different parties.

A third reason for evaluating one's work is to enhance science, in that one can contribute to the testing and development of theories by examining them in the applied setting. This can be mutually beneficial, as laboratory researchers will want to know whether their theories are applicable to a range of 'real world' situations, while practitioners will be interested in trying out new ideas.

Evaluation may also serve 'negative' functions, such as postponing any real action on a problem. Everything can be put 'on hold' until the relevant evaluation has been conducted – an acceptable form of procrastination. There is also the danger that evaluators may be placed in a position where they are carrying the responsibility for decisions and changes to a service, when these more properly belong with managers and policy-makers.

A final reason for conducting evaluations is to achieve professional recognition. Those who evaluate their work tend to have higher prestige, and may be invited to present their work at conferences or may publish it in a journal. Simpson (1989) has reviewed a related function of evaluation in order to earn and promote a professional status for nurses. He suggests that research activity is central to nursing's claim to be considered a profession, but argues that for community psychiatric nursing at least, there is little evidence to date that it is sufficiently research-based to promote itself as a profession.

Measuring indirect work

Institutional and community systems

Some attention has already been accorded to the evaluation of systems, such as hospital wards, in Chapter 2. There I considered the *Ward Atmosphere Scale*, which could be used to help staff to clarify difficulties and then to evaluate changes intended to improve matters. An example of such changes was the provision of specialised training for nurses in a psychiatric day hospital, together with changes to the programme of client activities. These were associated with an improvement in the ward atmosphere and with better clinical outcomes. I will now consider some additional ways of measuring and evaluating this kind of systems level work.

Work through carers and other agencies

Perhaps the first level of indirect work is that which is conducted through relevant others, such as work done through the carers of clients which would otherwise require direct work involvement. Evaluation of such work can take the form of simple percentages, indicating the impact of a number of aspects of a service. An illustration of this is a community alcohol team, consisting of two community psychiatric nurses and a range of other disciplines (West and Spinks, 1988). They evaluated the success of the team in educating, supporting and consulting with people with alcohol-related difficulties. For example, one of their objectives was to involve friends and relatives in the helping process. In the six-month period evaluated, 42 per cent of clients were seen with their partner, while 30 per cent were seen with friends or relatives. An additional aspect of indirect work was involving and communicating with other agencies. In these respects, 33 per cent of clients were seen jointly with other agency staff (where another agency was closely involved), 46 per cent of clients were referred back to other agencies at case closure, while in 61 per cent of cases a letter was written to the referring agent after the first appointment.

Although straightforward, this information related directly to the team's objectives, and provides the basis for repeated assessments (for example, over 6 months of every year). This would let them know whether they were getting better at achieving their various objectives over time.

Other methods used to evaluate the effects of working through carers of elderly people have been summarised by Woods and Britton (1985). They include carers' questionnaire ratings of the helpfulness of educational and support sessions, and the consideration of the impact of such sessions on the carers' coping mechanisms and morale.

Work through modified care environments

An alternative to indirect work through carers is based on changing the care setting. The resettlement of long-stay psychiatric hospital clients in community homes represents a major recent example. A number of these homes have now been evaluated, most commonly in terms of broad 'quality of life' measures. One evaluation (Lehman *et al.*, 1986) assessed 191 clients by means of two structured interviews, one focusing on quality of life, the other on mental status. The former interview lasted about an hour and covered the clients' quality of life in eight areas, including their living situation, leisure activities and social relations. Each area was rated in terms of client satisfaction on a scale from one ('terrible') to seven ('delighted'). By means of these interviews, Lehman *et al.* (1986) were able to evaluate the success of community homes, finding evidence that they provided more favourable environments for the clients.

Although they used different measures and conducted their evaluation in the UK, Gibbons and Butler (1987) reached a similar conclusion to that of Lehman *et al.* (1986). In addition to interviews, Gibbons and Butler added direct observation to sample client behaviour in a psychiatric hospital, a district General Hospital, and subsequently a hostel in the community in which the clients were resettled. The observational data indicated that, amongst other things, the move to the hostel resulted in more time spent by the clients using community services such as the hairdresser, shops, cafe. In their interviews, the clients attributed their improved quality of life to the greater freedom, flexibility and informality of the hostel.

A third and final 'quality of life' example (Simpson *et al.*, 1989) involved a different measure, concerned with staff attitudes and practices. A questionnaire was used to gather data in relation to 28 items, with respondents scoring between zero (when a 'client orientated' answer was given) and two (for an 'institution-orientated' answer). The authors found that the hostel ward staff were more client orientated, in attitudes and practices, than staff in a group home and a hospital ward.

Table 10.1 *A summary of the* Patient Opinion Survey, *as used to evaluate the client's quality of life*

Factor	Example items
1. Fearfulness	Are patients on your ward frightened of the staff?
2. Isolation and apathy	Do you feel lonely here?
3. Lack of individualisation	Do the patients on your ward have a say in how the ward is run?
4. Unsatisfactory surroundings	Do you feel at home here?
5. Lack of autonomy	Are you kept busy even if you want to relax?
6. Unsatisfactory personal hygiene facilities	Are patients on your ward allowed to have a bath in private?
7. Lack of status and recognition	Do the nurses on your ward spend enough time talking with you?
8. Restrictions of actions	Can patients on your ward make a cup of tea whenever they want to?

A case study

To illustrate the use of quality of life measures, consider an example from the work of the ward manager featured in Chapter 6. He has evaluated the impact of the moves made by clients from the ward to houses in the hospital grounds by means of several measures. The one we discussed was the *Patient Opinion Survey* (Macdonald *et al.*, 1988), a 42-item, nurse-administered questionnaire. Each client answers 'yes' or 'no' to each question. In addition, there are two open-ended questions about the 'best' and 'worst' thing about their place of residence.

The *Patient Opinion Survey* (POS) yields results in terms of six quality of life factors, as set out in *Table 10.1*. The ward manager and his nursing colleagues have used the *POS* to evaluate the impact of the clients' resettlement by administering it before and after the moves. He has also found the *POS* to be a useful way of stimulating staff discussion of their practices, such as how restrictive some ward routines are towards the clients.

Work through modifying care practices

Moving staff and clients to hostels in the community has often been associated with improved quality of client care, as the above studies have illustrated. However, this does not necessarily follow, and since some clients will stay in hospital the challenge of improving care practices still remains. One successful illustration of this kind of indirect work has been provided by Lavender (1987). He designed a set of questionnaires which were used to feed back information to staff working on psychiatric rehabilitation wards. Called the *Model Standards Questionnaires*, they covered the areas set out in *Table 10.2*.

The questionnaires were administered to the multidisciplinary teams of 12 wards by two members of the rehabilitation committee, which included nurses of all grades. Once summarised, the information from

Table 10.2. The Model Standards Questionnaire *used to improve the quality of care in psychiatric rehabilitation (Lavender, 1987)*

Questionnaire	Content
1. Individual programmes of treatment and care	10 items assessing the extent to which clients were engaged in particular therapeutic activities (for example personal hygiene; leisure skills). Scored between 1 and 10, based on the percentage of clients engaged in each activity.
2. Ward management practices	25 items gauging the extent to which clients were given autonomy, had their own personal possessions, and the social distance between staff and clients was minimised (for example, operating TV controls; own books and records). Scored by rating each management practice between 1 and 5.
3. Community contact practices	13 items concerning contacts between clients and community-based facilities. Scored in terms of the percentage of clients engaged in each particular type of community contact (1 to 10 scale).

two of the questionnaires was fed back to each ward as a series of specific recommendations concerning care practices. Nine months later the questionnaires were re-administered to assess changes in these care practices. By withholding information from one questionnaire for each ward, Lavender (1987) was able to control for the effects of feedback across all 12 wards. Also, by comparing scores before and after feedback, he was able to assess the impact of the information from the questionnaires. Finally, he assessed other possible explanations for any obtained changes, such as alterations in the nurse:client ratios and the involvement of other professional staff in therapies.

The results indicated that only the feedback from the *Individual Programmes of Treatment and Care Questionnaire* led to any improvement in care practices. Although there were trends for improvements in terms of the two other model standards questionnaires, these effects were not as strong.

This project illustrates the use of evaluation in developing a service, as discussed in the first section of this chapter. It also shows how care can be improved without any intervention in the traditional sense of the term. Simply providing good quality information (that is, specific and speedy) can achieve the kinds of results normally associated with major training or management changes. This reflects what often happens in direct work, when clients can improve because they receive accurate information about themselves, the so-called *baseline cure*.

Quality assurance

A popular example of such information based systems is Quality Assurance (QA), which has been hailed as a 'new frontier' in nursing (Lees *et al.*, 1987). These authors suggest that although QA consists of diverse ideas and practices, in essence it involves setting and pursuing professional standards of nursing care. Key dimensions are:

- accessibility of services
- appropriateness or relevance of the care that is provided
- effectiveness
- equity: that is, fair distribution of services to those with a need
- acceptability of client satisfaction – services should meet reasonable expectations; and
- efficiency: the service is economical (after Maxwell (1984)).

These dimensions reflect the elements of the nursing process, so QA should not be alien to nurses. Indeed, as Maxwell (1984) points out, Florence Nightingale is an impressive figure in the annals of QA because of her exposure of low standards of medical care in the army during the Crimean war. She also developed a system of hospital statistics which anticipated *performance indicators* (that is, basic information which allows comparisons to be made between services in different Districts, such as the number of client contacts per CPN per month).

In a survey of psychiatric day hospitals for elderly people (Milne and Drummond, 1990) we found evidence that nurses were pursuing the traditions of Florence Nightingale. Based on a structured interview with nursing staff, it appeared that the ten day-units we surveyed had developed good QA practices. These included accessible, equitable and acceptable services. However, it seemed that these nurses had evolved QA parallel to the general management initiative, rather than as a consequence of it. For instance, the nurses had not received any specific QA training, nor had they received management support. These findings raise questions about the relationship between QA and prior notions of good nursing practice, suggesting that QA may largely be a new term rather than a new idea. The exception we found to this lay in the area of evaluation, where the surveyed units were decidedly weak.

Social support

In Chapter 8 social support was defined in terms of informal help such as giving information, practical assistance, and emotional support. A questionnaire measure of social support, the *Inventory of Socially Supportive Behavior* (*ISSB*), was also introduced as an exercise in Chapter 2. In this section, I will summarise two additional measures and consider how they may contribute to the evaluation of indirect work, for example helping the carers of elderly dependents.

The *ISSB* records how frequently a client experiences certain kinds of help. Measuring social support in this way can produce a very misleading picture, as it fails to take into account how adequate or satisfactory that support is. For example, one client may have very few socially supportive interactions yet, because of their needs, feel highly satisfied with the support they receive. A second individual may have frequent and widespread support, yet feel that it is highly unsatisfactory in relation to their needs. For this reason, Krause and Markides (1990) altered the *ISSB* by adding a question about whether the clients were satisfied with the support that they received, and whether they wished it was provided more or less often. This question was raised for each of the four main types of social support ('informational', 'tangible', 'emotional' and 'integration'). The latter refers to the extent that clients provide support to others (for example, one item concerns whether someone 'depended on you for guidance and advice'). In a random community survey of 351 elderly people, the authors found evidence that all four types of support, and the respondents' satisfaction with these forms of support, served to buffer the impact of bereavement on depression.

Two further refinements of social support measures over the *ISSB* are contained in the *Significant Others Scale* (*SOS*; Power *et al.*, 1988). This requires the client to relate the types of support they receive to specific people in their social network. The client is asked to rate (on a one to seven scale) the extent to which they can 'trust, talk to frankly and share feelings with' a spouse or partner and other key people. In the second refinement, two versions of the form were used, one completed in relation to the 'actual' nature of help, and the second to measure the 'ideal' kind of support.

Power *et al.*'s (1988) results indicated that the *SOS* provided a good measure of the perceived provision of social support in a range of significant relationships. Of particular interest to mental health nurses is that the *SOS*'s real–ideal scores provide a basis for judging a client's need for social support.

Exercise 10.1: Observing social support

The two social support measures just mentioned are both set out as self-report questionnaires. One can think of situations in which this format would limit their use, for example with a client with poor eyesight, speech, or reading ability. Assuming such a difficulty, try to design a social support measure which could be based on direct observation of a client's behaviour. Perhaps making use of the headings of the *Inventory of Socially Supportive Behavior* in Chapter 2, set out a form which would allow you to record the relevant client behaviour by systematic observation. You may also be able to pilot the form with a client or a colleague. For example, you might set the main things you want to observe down the left hand column of a blank sheet of paper, then draw a series of vertical lines on the remainder of the sheet. These could be columns for time-sampling (for example, observing the amount of social support for five minutes of every hour).

A case study

The ward manager and nurses of a day unit for elderly people provide support, respite and advice to their clients' carers. To evaluate the service they have used a questionnaire which addressed such issues as the amount and appropriateness of the help provided, and this was posted to carers. But the ward manager found it to be redundant as the carers simply said that they felt perfectly able to let her know how well the service was working by means of phone calls or when meeting her on the day unit. She has therefore tended to rely on these 'spontaneous evaluations' as a guide for her indirect work.

Carers' comments on the respite service, for instance, have noted that the dependents' clothes had not all been returned; that they came home unclean; and that they had been 'pestered' by other clients while in the unit. In relation to home visits, the ward manager has the evidence of continued requests by carers to talk through their experience of caring, sometimes lasting after the death of their dependent. In addition to these spoken or overt forms of feedback on their work, the nurses ask the carers to keep a diary, to note whether there are any behaviour problems, whether medication has been taken and so on.

From these information sources, and her own observations (for instance, how well a carer is managing to keep the home organised) the ward manager is able to evaluate her work and see ways of improving it still further. Indeed, the diary is an example of a measure taken to improve communication, having realised that this was poor. As a second example, the ward manager had also learnt from working on communication with carers that this led to an increased demand for respite care and the other services, such as advice and support, provided in the community.

This illustration of evaluation shows some of the ways in which an informal approach can reap better dividends than one based on questionnaires and other sophisticated instruments. This approach still allows this experienced nurse to gather information on thoughts, feelings and behaviours in a range of ways and in a systematic manner. This is sufficient to permit her to make the indicated changes to the way she and her colleagues work, thus improving their work in their future.

Training

Logically, the range of evaluation measures in training should match the range of training goals: for every common goal, a measure should be available. In the simple sense that training is directed typically at improving skills, knowledge and attitudes, this match does exist. But the kind of specific goals that can be distinguished for workshops and so forth cannot be matched up readily to available measures. Such goals, would, for example, reflect those set out in *Table 5.1*, from Bloom's taxonomy of educational objectives. That table considers the cognitive or 'knowledge' domain, breaking it down into six levels of knowing, from awareness of facts to 'evaluation'. Each of these six levels might be the goal of a training endeavour, and hence suitable measures of the extent to which the goal was achieved would need to be found or devised in order to evaluate the training. Similarly the domains of skills and attitudes can be subdivided and targeted for training work.

In addition to the need to evaluate the thoughts, feelings and behaviours of the workshop participants, there is also a logical requirement to consider the impact of training on other related people. Referring back to Chapter 5, there is often interest in evaluating training in relation to the triadic model of trainer, mediator (who receives the training) and client. However, many workshop evaluations focus purely on the effect of training staff in terms of the benefits to their clients: there may be no evaluation of the staff's learning as such.

Finally, for each person in the triadic model some attention should be accorded to the ways in which the effects of training generalise. This might be the way in which they extend from thoughts to behaviours; or the maintenance of a training effect over time (for example, how attitudes have changed six months after a workshop); or finally the way in which those who have had training apply it in different places, to different people, and to different problems.

Thus, a truly comprehensive evaluation of training would consider the learning of the trainer, mediator and client; it would take account of the triple response system of thoughts, feelings and behaviours; and it would look for generalisation of the training across time, people, behaviours and settings.

Although the range of readily available measures does not match these logical requirements, there is still a considerable variety of interesting and practical instruments to consider. In addition, valuable measures can be based on simple, 'purpose-made' records of what people do, think or feel before and after training, as well as of generalisation.

Evaluating behaviour

Perhaps the domain in which there is the greatest number and range of accessible published measures is that of behaviour change. This is presumably because workshops intended to help people to acquire or enhance relevant skills are the most common form of training. In order to consider examples of measures, I will group them in terms of the way in which the skills were sampled.

The most direct and valid measure of training in skills is administered while the skill is being applied in routine client work. One example which has already been discussed is the *Helper Behaviour Rating System* (*HBRS*, Hardy and Shapiro, 1985: see *Table 6.1*). This allows the trainer to evaluate the effectiveness of training in 'prescriptive' and 'exploratory' forms of psychotherapy.

Less sophisticated measures have focused on a few key behaviours, as in the *Behaviour Therapy Proficiency Scale* (*BTPS*, Milne, 1986) which was used to evaluate a one-week workshop in behaviour therapy for psychiatric nurses. The *BTPS* covers five topics, including providing prompts and reinforcements to the client. Each nurse who attended the workshop was observed conducting a care plan and ratings were made. This yielded a score between zero and three for each of the five topics. In order to evaluate the workshop, comparisons were made on the *BTPS* with a control group. This suggested that the workshop was effective in developing the nurses' ability to conduct behavioural care plans. Another approach within direct observation is to evaluate general staff–client interactions, as in observing what goes on in a day room when nurses and clients are present. In Paul and Lentz's (1977) extensive evaluation of a psychiatric rehabilitation programme, these interactions were coded by means of the *Staff–resident Interaction Chronograph*. This notes five classes of client behaviour (such as 'inappropriate crazy') in relation to 21 classes of nurse behaviour (such as ignoring the client's behaviour), thus providing a very thorough evaluation.

A step removed from the direct observation of routine work as a means of skills evaluation is the use of role-plays or other simulations. Paxton *et al.* (1988) provided an example based on teaching student mental health nurses to use the conversational model of psychotherapy. They asked these nurses to role-play client and therapist, recording the interviews on audiotape before transcribing and analysing what the student 'therapists' said. An experimental group of students then received a two-day training in the conversational model of therapy, while their colleagues formed a control group. The interview was then repeated for both groups, and the data analysed in relation to 12 kinds of speech used by the student therapists. These included use of 'I and we', making 'statements not questions', 'negotiation' and offering 'understanding hypotheses'. Significant increases were obtained in these categories for the experimental group, but for all but the 'statements not questions' category this was also true for the control group. Paxton *et al.* (1988) suggested that the reason for this outcome was that the experimental group had informally taught their colleagues in the control group about the model of therapy (that is, they were so enthused by it that they unconsciously modelled the key behaviours). Although this represents a problem with the design of the evaluation, it also illustrates generalisation across people, or what has been called *pyramid training*: Paxton *et al.* (1988) seemed to have discovered a quick and easy way of extending the effects of their training!

A further step removed from directly observing the impact of training on behaviour are evaluation devices such as simulations and critical incidents. These analogues can take the form of live or video demonstrations to which the 'trainee' makes a written response. This would typically be between different courses of action. To illustrate, Flanagan *et al.* (1979), in training parents to use a behavioural technique ('time-out'), used a 12-item audiotape which presented

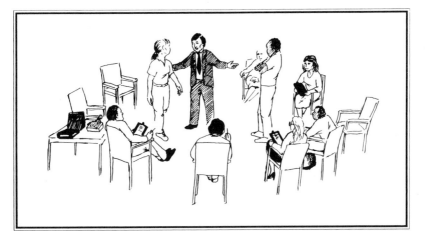

Role-playing

examples of typical situations requiring the use of 'time-out'. The parents were asked to choose amongst several ways of responding to the child, only one of which was 'correct'. For example, normally such tests give credit for sending the child to a non-reinforcing place (such as the corner of a room) immediately following an undesirable behaviour.

Perhaps a final step removed are those measures which are purely paper and pencil tasks, such as writing down how you would formulate or tackle a problem. At this stage, the measures are probably evaluating thinking rather than gauging behaviour, so I will address them next.

Evaluating thinking

In Chapter 4 I discussed the triple response system of thoughts, feelings and behaviours, noting that there may at times be considerable overlap or *synchrony*. Perhaps because of this phenomenon, some evaluators only measure one form of response and assume parallel changes in the remaining two. As in the case of client change, the evidence from training would suggest that there can be *desynchrony* between the different types of response, and hence it is unwise to make this assumption.

A classic example of this is Gardner's (1972) study of the effectiveness of two different training methods – education role-plays and lectures – provided to two groups of nurses. Measures of knowledge and skills were administered before and after each method of training. The knowledge measure consisted of a 229-item questionnaire in a True/False format, while behaviour change was observed directly in work with clients. Gardner found that the role-play based learning only led to changes in behaviour, while the lectures only led to improvements in knowledge. This type of association between a training method and a specific kind of learning has been reported by other researchers.

An alternative to the questionnaire as a measure of knowledge is the unstructured assessment method, in which the recipient of training is asked to write down what they would do in relation to critical incidents. Milne and Whyke (1988), for example, developed a measure of a nursing care plan, which was written by nurses before and after the ENB 953 course (*Developments in psychiatric nursing*). The nurses were given four blank pages and asked to:

> Select a client from your current clinical area. Write a nursing care plan detailing the care of this client. Please spend around 30 minutes on the care study. The aim of the exercise is to produce the main ideas, headings, procedures, etc., that you would wish to use.

A detailed scoring key was designed to assess the nurses' replies, giving credit for appropriate information in eight categories (for example, the use of a nursing model). It was found that the nurses in this study obtained significantly higher scores on this measure for three out of the eight categories following training.

Evaluating attitudes

The conventional way to assess changes in the 'feeling' domain is by considering the attitudes of those receiving training. The attitudes may be towards the topic covered in training (for example, nursing models), towards the client group intended to benefit from the training (for example, the elderly), or may focus on a general disposition amongst those receiving training (such as attitude to psychotherapy).

As an example of the latter, consider the *Conservatism Scale* (Wilson and Patterson, 1968). This is designed to measure a flexible, non-authoritarian approach to clients. It consists of 100 items, and staff reply whether they believe in, or are in favour of them. Items include straitjackets, divorce and royalty.

To examine attitudes towards the topic of training, there is an *Attitude to Treatment Questionnaire* (*ATQ*: Caine and Smail, 1968) which consists of 40 items in the form of statements, responded to by one of five options, ranging from strongly agree to strongly disagree. Items include 'nurse–patient relationships can be just as effective in treatment as doctor–patient relationships'; and 'by and large, psychotherapy is a waste of time'. The *ATQ* would therefore measure attitudes towards psychotherapy.

I have used both the *ATQ* and the conservatism scale as part of the evaluation of the one-week workshop in behaviour therapy for mental health nurses, as mentioned earlier (Milne, 1986). Significant improvements were obtained in terms of skill and knowledge measures, but there was little evidence of change on either of these attitude instruments. This was, therefore, evidence of desynchrony in the triple response system, begging questions about the importance of attitude change in training of this kind. That is, if training produces changes in the skills and knowledge that nurses bring to bear in their work with clients, and these produce better clinical results (as we found), then what importance have attitudes?

One answer appears to be that they effect the motivation to make use of training. Those who have unfavourable attitudes towards an intervention or a client group may still do good work. However, they may do it less frequently than those whose attitudes are more favourable. This point may recall the one made in favour of *acceptability* or *consumer satisfaction* ratings in the preceding chapter, namely that acceptability can be seen as an important determinant of the use of a service. Such ratings also provide a unique perspective, and so enhance an evaluation. In terms of training, acceptability ratings can be regarded as a form of attitude evaluation in the sense of being a measure of the mediators' feelings about the training they have received. To illustrate, the nurse therapist course run at Moorhaven Hospital, Devon, made use of eight-point rating scales (ranging from 'very poor' to 'excellent') to obtain acceptability ratings on five areas of the course, including 'theoretical instruction', 'clinical experience' and a general course evaluation.

Turning to the third example, there are also instruments for measuring attitudes towards client groups and to working with them. Snape (1986), for instance, enquired into nurses' attitudes towards care of the elderly, as there were difficulties in recruiting staff to the relevant wards. A 30-item attitude scale was developed, based on the same five-point ratings as the *Attitude to Treatment Questionnaire*. Items included:

- elderly patients are uninteresting to nurses;
- people should be thoroughly medically investigated, even when old;
- what the doctor says goes in the management of elderly patients.

Turning to attitudes towards the client group, Doka (1986) studied the perceptions of older people held by adolescents. He used a *sentence completion* approach, in which the youths were asked to complete such sentences as: 'Most 75-year-olds are . . .'. Their replies were coded as positive (for example, completing the sentence with 'kind'), negative (for example, 'cranky'), or neutral (for example, 'grey haired'). Doka reported that the adolescents' attitudes towards elderly people became more negative as the age of the person they were rating increased.

A case study

I spoke with two post-basic nurse tutors whose job included assessing learning needs, providing workshops and evaluating their impact for nurses in a large psychiatric hospital. They outlined several different measures of the training they provide. The one that caught my imagination was an open-ended questionnaire which they had used recently to evaluate a Quality Assurance (QA) workshop. The workshop had focused on areas of practice that need QA measures and the related question of standard setting. It had been attended by a multidisciplinary audience of staff working in the mental health unit. What appealed to me about the questionnaire was that it used the main concepts of QA to evaluate the training in QA, that is, it was a *reflexive* or internally consistent way to conduct the evaluation. *Table 10.3* sets out the tutors' form, together with some of the comments they received back from the workshop participants.

The questionnaire was completed after the workshop and the information was used for several purposes. It was summarised and fed back to the hospital's QA group (the workshop organisers) to act as a guide for any future events. The tutors also felt that such evaluations helped them to justify some events (for instance, to sceptical managers); it provided an indication of the attenders' current interests and concerns; and, in the case of QA at least, it demonstrated that they 'practised what they preached' by evaluating what they did, after having encouraged others to evaluate their own work. This also indicated reflexivity in the evaluation process, to complement that in the questionnaire's structure.

The two tutors also had reservations about evaluating their training, however. One (which arose with the QA event) was that only a minority of forms may be returned, inevitably giving a biased picture. A related difficulty has been the diversity of the feedback which they do receive. On one hand, different attenders can provide diametrically opposed comments; on the other, the tutors' own perceptions may be at variance with the feedback. Under such circumstances it is difficult to know which evidence to note. For example, the tutors know from experience that attenders can be very dissatisfied with role-plays, yet acknowledge learning a great deal from them. (This is another instance of desynchrony in outcomes, with an affective measure suggesting a poor result, and a cognitive one indicating the opposite).

The tutors tend to consider a range of such outcomes when they evaluate training, including the development of more realistic goal-

Table 10.3 *The* QA Workshop Evaluation Questionnaire, *with a selection of the participants' comments*

We would be very grateful for any comments you may have concerning the quality of today's workshop. We are interested in how valuable the day was for you, whether you enjoyed it, its relevance to your work, in fact, anything that you care to mention! Signatures are, of course, optional.

Structure (for example plan of workshop, organisation, time allocated to different subjects etc)
- 'very flexible plan, which partly threw me as I like to stick to the timetable'
- 'workable numbers and appropriate group sizes; space good'
- 'content interesting and applicable'

Process (for example nature of teaching, flexibility of approach, support, etc)
- 'great deal of support'
- 'time wasted getting groups together: guidelines would help'
- 'provoked discussion and involvement'

Outcome (for example results, opinions, comments)
- 'ultimate aim was achieved: participants appeared to understand how to set standards'
- 'feel I know more than I did at the beginning'
- 'clarified thought about the subject'

Overall comments
- 'most educative and enjoyable'
- 'a day worth doing: momentum re-established'
- 'made the task (implementing QA) seem more achievable'

setting skills, reappraised attitudes, and awareness of new developments. This represents an interest in behaviours, feelings and thoughts, as stressed earlier in this section. They recognise that it is important to evaluate the generalisation of training (from workshop to workplace) but they rarely find the time to undertake this level of evaluation.

Summary

Evaluation can be seen to serve a range of functions, the most acclaimed of which is to provide systematic feedback to a service or unit. This affords a logical basis on which to make corrective changes, thus improving the service over time. In order for the evaluation to be useful it is necessary to use sound and appropriate measures (as well as good research designs, as set out in Chapter 9). Examples are offered from three forms of indirect work: training, social support and systems-level intervention (for example, 'quality of life' analysis). Case study material illustrates some of the main points of the chapter and indicates that evaluation is a strong feature in the work of some mental health nurses. They provide good models of research-based nursing practice.

Questions for further consideration

1 At the start of the chapter I emphasised some of the reasons why staff evaluate services. Try to set out some reasons why they do *not* evaluate more often than they do. This should help to develop your understanding of the many factors which influence evaluation.

2 The evaluation of training can become a major undertaking. What do you regard as the appropriate kind of evaluation for the following forms of training? Try to justify your answers:
   a) a two-hour seminar on 'nursing standards';
   b) a one-day workshop for carers of elderly people;
   c) a two-day workshop for nursing staff on continence promotion;
   d) a series of six half-hour talks to GPs on the nature of the CPN service.

3 Think of an example where some training that you received made its impact across the 'triple response system' (that is, your thoughts, feelings and behaviour). Can you think of a way to measure this effect?

4 Can 'quality of life' ever be measured adequately by quantitative methods (such as questionnaires)? How else might it be assessed? What are the strengths and weaknesses of these options?

5 At several points in the chapter I have highlighted evidence that the feedback of information may constitute a powerful 'intervention' into a system. Can you think of a setting in which you have worked recently where a specific form of feedback would be beneficial? Try to set this out as if it were a detailed proposal to the manager concerned.

References

Brooker, C. G. D. and Simmons, S. M. (1985). A study to compare two models of community psychiatric nursing care delivery. *Journal of Advanced Nursing, 10,* 217–223.

Caine, T. M. and Smail, D. J. (1968). Attitudes of psychiatric nurses to their role in treatment. *British Journal of Medical Psychology, 41*, 193–197.

Campbell, D. T. and Stanley, J. C. (1963). *Experimental and quasi-experimental designs for research*. Chicago: Rand McNally.

Doka, K. J. (1986). Adolescent attitudes and beliefs toward ageing and the elderly. *International Journal of Ageing and Human Development, 22*, 173–187.

Flanagan, S., Adams, H. E. and Forehand, R. (1979). A comparison of four instrumental techniques for teaching parents to use time out. *Behaviour Therapy, 10*, 94–102.

Gardner, J. M. (1972). Teaching behaviour modification to non-professionals. *Journal of Applied Behaviour Analysis, 5*, 517–521.

Gibbons, J. S. and Butler, J. P. (1987). Quality of life of new long stay psychiatric in-patients: the effects of moving to a hostel. *British Journal of Psychiatry, 151*, 347–354.

Hardy, G. E. and Shapiro, D. A. (1985). Therapist response modes in prescriptive vs exploratory psychotherapy. *British Journal of Clinical Psychology, 24*, 235–245.

Hersen, M. and Barlow, D. H. (1976). *Single Care Experimental Designs*. Oxford: Pergamon.

Krause, N. and Markides, K. (1990). Measuring social support among older adults. *International Journal of Ageing and Human Development, 30*, 37–53.

Lavender, A. (1987). Improving the quality of care on psychiatric rehabilitation wards: a controlled evaluation. *British Journal of Psychiatry, 150*, 476–481.

Lees, G. D., Richman, J., Salauroo, M. A. and Warden, S. (1987). Quality assurance: is it professional insurance? *Journal of Advanced Nursing, 12*, 719–727.

Lehman, A. F., Possidente, S. and Hawker, F. (1986). The quality of life of chronic patients in a state hospital and in community residences. *Hospital and Community Psychiatry, 37*, 901–907.

MacDonald, L., Sibbald, B. and Hoare, C. (1988). Measuring patient satisfaction with life in a long-stay psychiatric hospital. *The International Journal of Social Psychiatry, 34*, 292–304.

Marks, I. M. (1985). *Psychiatric Nurse Therapists in Primary Care*. London: Royal College of Nursing.

Maxwell, R. J. (1984). Quality assessment in health. *British Medical Journal, 288*, 1470–1472.

Milne, D. L. (1986). *Training Behaviour Therapists: Methods, Evaluation and Implementation with Parents, Nurses and Teachers*. London: Croom Helm.

Milne, D. L. and Drummond, R. (1990). Quality Assurance: A survey of nursing practice. *International Journal of Health Care Quality Assurance, 3*, 16–18.

Milne, D. L. and Whyke, T. (1988). New measures for the formative and summative evaluation of a post-basic psychiatric nursing education course. *Journal of Advanced Nursing, 13*, 79–86.

Paul, G. L. and Lentz, R. J. (1977). *Psychosocial Treatment of Chronic Mental Patients: Milieu versus Social Learning Programmes*. Cambridge, Massachusetts: Harvard University Press.

Paxton, R., Rhodes, D. and Crooks, I. (1988). Teaching nurses therapeutic conversation: a pilot study. *Journal of Advanced Nursing, 13*, 401–404.

Power, M. J., Champion, L. A. and Aris, S. J. (1988). The development of a measure of social support: the Significant Others (SOS) Scale. *British Journal of Clinical Psychology, 27*, 349–358.

Simpson, C. J., Hyde, C. E. and Faragher, E. B. (1989). The chronically mentally ill in community facilities: a study of quality of life. *British Journal of Psychiatry, 154,* 77–82.

Simpson, K. (1989). Community Psychiatric Nursing: a research-based profession? *Journal of Advanced Nursing, 14,* 274–280.

Snape, J. (1986). Nurses' attitudes to care of the elderly. *Journal of Advanced Nursing, II,* 569–572.

West, J. and Spinks, P. (Eds; 1988). *Clinical Psychology in Action.* London: Wright.

Wilson, G. D. and Patterson, J. R. (1968). A new measure of conservatism. *British Journal of Social and Clinical Psychology, 7,* 264–269.

Woods, R. T. and Britton, P. G. (1985). *Clinical Psychology with the Elderly.* London: Routledge.

Further reading

Baldwin, S., Godfrey, C. and Propper, C. (Eds; 1990). *Quality of Life: Perspectives & Policies:* London: Routledge.
This recent book looks at different theories, methods and evaluations of 'quality of life'. Amongst other contributions, there are chapters on how to measure quality of life and an examination of it in relation to spouse carers.

Evaluation and Program Planning (1987) 10:3.
This Pergamon journal produced a special issue on 'simple measures' used in mental health services. The editors' aims were to encourage the use of simple measures and to promote their appropriate application. They argued that such simple measures, if correctly used, can provide very helpful information on services. Examples from this issue included measures of acceptability, outcome, process and quality assurance. In general, the journal is a rich source of applicable ideas and instruments.

Faulkner, A. (1985). The evaluation of teaching interpersonal skills to nurses. In C. M. Kagan (Ed.) *Interpersonal Skills in Nursing.* London: Croom Helm.
This chapter considers some of the difficulties in measuring nursing skills before moving on to argue the need for a baseline assessment and to provide examples of relevant measures.

Milne, D. (1986). *Training Behaviour Therapists: Methods, Evaluation and Implementation with Parents, Nurses and Teachers.* London: Routledge.
As reflected by the emphasis given in this chapter, I consider training to be of major importance. Of particular concern in the above book is the relationship between how we train and its impact on what is learned and applied in one's work. Literature reviews and three extensive 'case studies' are used to deal with these issues. Perhaps the most unusual feature of the book lies in its attention to the evaluation of training, in the broad way outlined in this chapter. Do not be put off by the title: the material that is reviewed will prove of interest to anyone with a concern for effective training.

Reid, E. (1988). An overview of quality assurance – the concept and the reality. *Recent Advances in Nursing, 19,* 64–97.
This is a broad, very well referenced and helpful summary of various aspects of QA and related concepts. These include 'performance indicators', 'quality circles', 'nursing standards', 'qualpacs' and more! An excellent introduction to terms and their origins.

SECTION SIX

Conclusion

11 Themes and implications

I began this book with an acknowledgement that it would prove difficult to do justice to the scope of psychology, but with the view that much of value could still be discussed. In trying to summarise what has been discussed, three themes emerge. They concern the importance of a problem-solving approach, the context of mental health nursing and the nature of nursing.

The problem-solving approach

The nursing process is a problem-solving blend of assessment, planning, intervention and evaluation. As far as direct clinical work is concerned, this provides a coherent and rational approach. In addition, one theme running throughout this book is that it also provides the basis for a scientific approach in mental health nursing. This emerges partly from the explicitly experimental nature of the nursing process – that is, adapting the care plan in the light of the evaluation evidence. As Ward (1985) put it:

> . . . conclusions about the choice of care should all be derived through careful observation and analysis, and the final selection of the care alternatives derived from (these) studies (p19).

This is the language of science, of 'knowledgeable doers'. It encourages a scientific approach to one's work. The obvious contrast is with the uncritical, routine and undiscriminating use of techniques, where clients receive similar 'packages' of care regardless of their individual needs, while the impact of these techniques is not evaluated. This not only prevents progress, but also fosters a negative attitude towards knowledge and experimentation. Thus, a problem-solving approach, such as the nursing process, carries with it positive implications for theory and practice.

The second sense in which the nursing process paves the way for a more scientific approach is by emphasising and enhancing evaluation skills. It is one thing to have a repertoire of highly-polished clinical skills which are perhaps very relevant to current practices or settings. It is quite another to develop new ones to meet new challenges, as illustrated by the nurse whose ward closes down and who has to adapt to work in a community hostel. For this transition to be a success, a number of ingredients are important, including adequate management and training. However, there is a definite limit to the scope of these ingredients as, for example, each of the above would tend to offer only general solutions. The vital missing ingredient is the capacity to learn and adapt to such new challenges by means of careful, locally-focused evaluations. As stressed throughout the text (and especially in the preceding two chapters), evaluation can provide feedback, from which one learns how to do a better job. The nursing process can provide this feedback, indicating which skills are still valid and which require modification. The key skill in this situation, therefore, lies in designing evaluations which will generate the best possible feedback.

The exercise of this skill, therefore, has profound implications in terms of shaping the future of mental health nursing. An analogy can be drawn with grapes, as, like the nursing process, they contain all the ingredients needed to become something special, in this case, wine! All that is required are the correct conditions, which in nursing includes the problem-solving approach.

Example: evaluations of nurse therapy

I would like to review the example of the nurse behaviour therapist in order to illustrate the importance of evaluation. Training in behaviour therapy was initially provided to five experienced nurses over a three year period by Marks and colleagues (1977), in London, yielding promising results. Since then Marks and his colleagues have conducted a series of evaluations, which have helped to define this developing role for nurses.

The initial evaluation indicated that nurse behaviour therapists could achieve clinical outcomes which were comparable to those obtained by other professional groups (Marks *et al.*, 1977). Ginsberg and Marks (1977) also studied the cost benefits of nurse therapy, considering the extent to which 42 clients used health care resources before and after therapy. Large changes were reported in such areas as the number of in-patient weeks (88 per cent reduction) and GP help (59 per cent reduction). Subsequently, Marks (1985) has evaluated the effectiveness of nurse therapists in primary care, in comparison to routine GP management, again obtaining positive results. These included clinical outcomes for the mainly phobic disorders, together with the client's opinions and another cost-benefit analysis. Outcomes were compared after one year, and it was found that those clients who were helped by the nurse therapist improved markedly, whereas those seen by their GPs had changed little. The clients preferred the new health centre service to attendance at out-patient settings, while the costs of health care resources decreased slightly for the nurse therapy clients, but increased in the case of the control group (the GPs' clients).

The example of nurse therapy shows how evaluation, an essential element in any problem-solving approach, goes hand-in-hand with developments in nursing. Such evaluations help to clarify what nurses offer in relation to other professionals, as well as providing a firm basis from which to argue for increases in numbers or alterations to services. To illustrate, Paykel and Griffith (1983) were able to conclude, from their comparison of CPN care with out-patient care from psychiatrists, that it was equally effective, cost less and produced higher client satisfaction. They then went on to argue for an extension of this kind of CPN service.

The context of mental health nursing

A second major theme throughout this book has been the importance of understanding events in their context. A range of illustrations was provided in Chapter 2, and other chapters have continued the emphasis in relation to the different elements of the nursing process. It has also been recognised that events can provide a context for developments in nursing, as in politically-inspired policies of 'community care' or professionally-led reappraisals of the nurse's role. Events and contexts therefore interact, in the sense that it is difficult to adequately understand the one without reference to the other.

Thus, Walton (1986) suggested that the nursing process emerged in the context of professional concerns to:

- identify and clarify the role of the nurse;
- achieve professional status for nursing and its acceptance as an academic discipline;
- counteract falling standards of care and attendant decline in job satisfaction;
- narrow the gap between theory and reality in education; and
- re-establish the centrality of the clinical nursing role.

Similarly, the policy of 'community care' in the UK can be understood in the context of the government's self-help ideology, its concern over expenditure, a need to implement general management, and so forth.

The implications of this view include the way in which we can better understand events (including client behaviour) by considering their context, and the role that can then be played in shaping them. Because of its growing importance, and its emphasis in Project 2000, I would like to consider 'prevention' as a case in point. How can we use this 'contextual' view to make sense of preventative care? And what should nurses be doing as a result?

Example: prevention

Prevention means stopping something from happening, but in the mental health field this is by no means as clear or as straightforward as it might seem. Caplan (1964), for instance, has noted three different stages of 'prevention', namely *primary* (stopping people showing the first signs of a health problem), *secondary* (stopping initial signs of difficulty progressing to more serious forms) and *tertiary* prevention (stopping those with significant difficulties becoming incapacitated). In addition, as Newton (1988) states, there are obstacles to defining the mental health problem, identifying its cause, and in finding ways to either eradicate the cause or 'fortify' the individual. Such obstacles, she points out, have dogged efforts at conceptualising, researching and implementing preventative measures for the 80 years since the 'Mental Hygiene' movement first began. Her book is an attempt to review and develop our understanding of prevention efforts since 1900.

A filter model

One illustration of these complexities is the way in which someone becomes a mental health service client. Goldberg and Huxley (1980) considered those factors which influenced a client's passage to in-patient psychiatric status, providing a model to summarise three stages or *filters* through which such a client passes. The first filter arose when a client decided to consult their GP, and at this stage the severity of the problem was one of the major determinants of whether they passed through to the next filter or not. The second filter concerned the GP's ability to recognise the problem, and here factors such as the frequency of surgery attendances by the client were important. Finally, referral to a psychiatrist (the third filter) was most likely to occur when the problem was a severe mental breakdown. Other factors, influential at all stages, included the client's age, marital status and educational level.

In addition to client factors, Goldberg and Huxley also found that characteristics of the doctor influenced the kind of care provided. A GP's ability to recognise a mental health problem, for example, will vary with his or her style of interviewing and knowledge base. They noted 10 such factors in the interview, all potentially amenable to improvement by training (for example, clarifying the presenting complaint and sensitivity to nonverbal cues). These findings indicate that even the detection of a mental health problem is a complex process, involving major contributions from the GP and the client.

The client's role

As a second illustration, consider the role played by the client in trying to 'prevent' progress through the mental health filters. In terms of the coping model, set out in Chapter 1, the client can influence the presentation of a problem by the way in which he or she perceives it. He or she can also attempt to control or reduce the problem by the use of personal coping strategies or by eliciting social support. Either approach can prevent them from reaching the first filter. For instance, a study by Hickey *et al.* (1988) considered such preventive health practices as information-seeking (for example, reading articles about health), risk-avoidance (for example, checking the home for hazards) and daily health routines (for example, exercise and regular meals).

In addition, it is recognised that life transitions can play a significant part in the presentation of a problem, in the sense that they can represent either an unbearable level of stress or a diminution of coping. A report from the Royal College of General Practitioners (1981) noted a range of psychosocial transitions across the age range. Thus, young adults are more likely to experience pregnancy and the loss of a parent, while older adults are prone to experiencing retirement, and the loss of physical functions.

The role of the environmental context

As already mentioned, the stressfulness of life events and impaired coping are exacerbated by such factors as low educational level or marital status. Additional factors, according to the Royal College of General Practitioners (1981) report, are low socio-economic status, having several young children at home, unemployment and over-crowded housing conditions. To these might be added the 'isms' (such as ageism, sexism and racism), the pollutants (such as noise, vibration, air), as well as difficulties over housing, finances, ill-health, relationships and so on.

Interactions between clients, GPs and environments

By definition, stressful contextual events are those which are experienced as difficult by the client, rather than being defined by some objective criteria. There follow, therefore, inevitable interactions between individuals and environments. The GP's perception of the situation, for example, will be coloured by such things as his or her training, motivation and resources. If there is time and willingness to conduct a thorough interview, and if the GP knows that services are readily available, then a mental health problem is more likely to be detected, diagnosed and referred on.

Clients, in turn, will vary in terms of their recognition and disclosure of a problem. Such factors as their capacity to suffer ('stoicism' or 'hardiness'), their history of similar difficulties in the past, and their expectations of future help may influence their presentation. Newton (1988) cites research suggesting that additional factors affecting the client's reaction to a stressful event include how well prepared he or she is, how much control he or she has, how great a threat is posed and the amount of life change that is indicated.

Three models

There are a number of different perspectives on prevention. Three prominent ones are the *developmental, personal resources* and *social structures* models (Newton, 1988). These are summarised in *Table 11.1*, together with the sorts of preventative actions which nurses might take.

In essence, all three models help us to understand prevention by giving a central role to coping as part of a complex of psychosocial stressors. The basic options available to nurses are to assist individuals to cope more effectively, either to alter as far as possible the stressors or

Table 11.1 *Three dominant models in the prevention of mental health problems, following Newton (1988), together with some nursing implications*

Prevention model	Some implications for mental health nursing
1. **Developmental** focus on the life history of 'high risk' individuals	• helping parents to cope with their children and related stressors (for example social isolation; low self-esteem) • reducing marital discord • strengthen the child's coping strategies/social support
2. **Personal resources** concentrate on how people cope (personal coping strategies and social support)	• developing personal coping strategies and improving social support amongst clients • assisting clients to reduce strain • offering practical help
3. **Social structures** examine how roles (for example parenting and working) influence stress and coping	• support in seeking employment or professional help • helping clients to re-appraise role relationships • preparing clients for stressful situations (for example information and social skills)

to adjust to them; to focus on those who because of their developmental history are 'at risk'; and to attempt to address the social
structures which contribute to mental health difficulties.

Implications

On the basis of these models, it can be seen that 'prevention' is far from
the simple, common sense thing it is sometimes portrayed as.
Furthermore, it is far from straightforward to address. However, as
Table 11.1 indicated, there is a range of positive actions that nurses (and
others) can take to promote a preventive approach in mental health
work. They can also consider new ways of allocating resources to
prevention and review traditional practices. To expand on the latter
point, more attention to preventive work implies changes in a nurse's
relationships with clients and with other professionals (for example,
working indirectly more of the time, and doing so in more diverse
ways). It also implies a re-conceptualisation of 'the problem', which for
some people means focusing efforts on 'social structures', including the
politics of such common stressors as poor housing and high unemployment (Bender, 1976). There are also implications for the way nurses
are trained, for their tolerance of role change, and for their relationships
with other professions.

In short, preventive work appears to be every bit as challenging as
the more familiar tasks of acute care and rehabilitation. Moreover, it is
new and different in some important respects, which probably explains
why relatively little practical work is undertaken. But there is also
much that is done, and much that is familiar. The most fundamental
point is that a client's difficulty has to be understood in its context.

The nature of nursing

In Chapter 1, I recorded the old and simple distinction between curing
and caring, in which the former was seen as the only interesting task.
This distinction is hard to maintain, as is evident from the social
support literature, and observations of interactions between the nurse
and client in hospitals. These findings indicate that the therapeutic
potential of different kinds of relationships is by no means straightforward. As Chapters 2 and 8 pointed out, those who occupy some of
the apparently neutral therapeutic roles in society (such as carers and
hairdressers) seem to provide important forms of psychological help.
'Curing' is therefore not the exclusive province of the mental health
professionals, nor can it always be attributed with confidence to
specific professional activities. Other examples are the kinds of 'inmate
coercion' processes which undermine so-called 'therapeutic regimes'

in institutions (see Chapter 2), and the obstinate difficulty of pinning down clear links between a therapy and a client's improvement (see Chapter 6). Some professional activities are even counter-therapeutic, such as prescribing tablets which make people worse (as some tranquilisers do); the term *iatrogenesis* is applied to this.

Similarly, the notion that 'caring' is a discrete category does not withstand close inspection. Like diagnostic terms such as 'depression', caring is multidimensional. It varies across people (professionals, non-professionals and dependents), as well as across time, place and so on. Thus, although nursing may well be regarded as the major caring profession (DHSS, 1972) it is clear that many others may also provide significant amounts and forms of 'caring' (defined by McFarlane, 1976, as having feelings of concern, of interest, of oversight with a view to protection towards clients). The most striking examples are found amongst the client's family and friends. Hall's (1990) review of 'caring' includes estimates that there are five million family 'carers' in the community in the UK, and that 25 per cent of all adults will be a carer at some time in their lives. But as McFarlane (1976) also notes, other professionals may also have a caring role, albeit less prominent than that in nursing.

Role prescriptions

McFarlane (1976) goes on to define nursing generally in terms of helping clients who are having difficulty with daily activities of living to resume an independent existence. This is done by means of assisting, guiding, teaching, supporting, serving and caring, through the application of the nursing process.

This sounds like an adequate definition until one considers who it excludes. A good definition would exclude all groups save nurses. But with the minor exception of the reference to the nursing process (which is, after all, a widely used problem-solving framework, known by other names), McFarlane's definition could apply to any professional group to a greater or lesser extent. It also applies to non-professional carers, although their dependants would not be referred to as 'clients'. Thus, barring some special terms, the definition seems too general to be satisfactory.

The acid test of a good definition which I find myself using is not just based on logic. It is the down-to-earth situation of justifying one's role to a sceptic, such as a general manager. Hard questions that do get asked include: 'Why do we need your profession?' What is your distinctive contribution?' These are the difficult, 'bottom-line' questions which McFarlane's (1976) definition might not answer satisfactorily.

How can a better reply be structured? Cormack (1983), in reviewing the definitions of the mental health nurse, noted that these are largely based on statements of what the nurse should be, so-called *prescriptions*. These included sociotherapeutic, psychotherapeutic and administrative roles. While interesting and potentially useful, in Cormack's opinion such prescriptions 'do not coincide . . . nurses do not appear to be doing what the literature suggests they ought to be doing' (p20).

Role descriptions

This suggests that one issue is the way in which the nurse's role is defined. Different approaches reveal different roles. This can be helpful when the basis for any role statement is clear (that is, prescription or description) since, for instance, it suggests professional objectives. But when the two are confused, problems can arise. For example, consider again the situation where one is describing one's role to a manager. In such a situation, combining prescriptions with descriptions might produce a rather grandiose account, one which overlapped unrealistic- ally with the roles of others or which was unattainable in practice. Thus, community psychiatric nurses might claim to specialise in community work with clients (for examples, their interactions with family members), although careful descriptions of their work indicate that social workers are more likely to fulfil this role (Wooff *et al.,* 1988). Similarly, they may claim that their work is research-based, while the evidence would suggest otherwise (Simpson, 1989). It is important to consider the implications of such public reputations of role prescriptions, as they may create a credibility gulf. Prescriptions therefore need to stay in touch with descriptions.

In addition to being clear about the prescriptive or descriptive basis for role statements, two further issues will help to structure a reply to my hypothetical manager. One is to provide a detailed account of what one does (or wishes to do), which I will call *elaboration*. The other is to take account of *motivation,,* that which one is encouraged to do.

Role elaboration

Nature hates a category! The reality in nature is that things are not simply black or white, but various shades of grey. This point was made in Chapter 1, in relation to diagnostic categories, and applies equally strongly to the ways in which we describe professional roles. In this sense, if we claim to provide care or counselling we fly in the face of nature, which would teach us that these are complex, variable phenomena.

In order to do them justice, one therefore needs to describe a role in terms of several dimensions. Counselling, for example, can reflect different therapeutic models and be practised with a range of competencies. It can vary in duration and scope, in its aims and content, counsellors can be more or less trained, and so on.

If one accepts this logic, the appropriate way to describe one's role is in terms of several dimensions. In *Figure 11.1*, I have set out an illustration in the form of a *role-profile*. The title indicates that a professional group or an individual will be represented by different points on each dimension, in relation to different tasks. This relates the nature of the work done to the quality with which it is pursued. A profile could be constructed prescriptively (for example, what your team or manager thought you should be doing) and/or descriptively (that is, based on some kind of record of what you actually did).

By elaborating the role statement in this fashion, communication difficulties due to category-type descriptions are minimised. One also explicitly recognises variability amongst members of the same and different professional groups. On this point, I would expect that this profile would become more and more discriminating between groups as one's sample increased. That is, some nurses will work in ways that are very similar to some social workers or some psychologists. But I doubt that this would be true for a sample of 50 members of each such

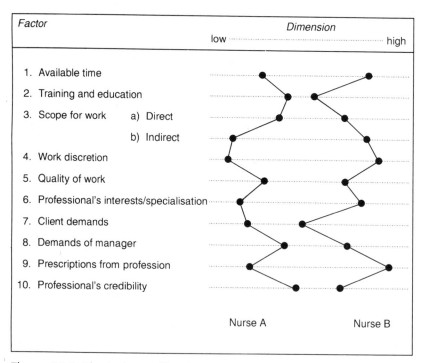

Figure 11.1 *The 'role-profile' – a way of defining professional roles in relation to specific tasks. Completed for two hypothetical nurses, A and B.*

group. In a practical vein, this sort of elaborate profile could greatly facilitate discussions of roles, for example, between team members. To illustrate, it would be unlikely that any one team would contain two members with identical descriptive or prescriptive profiles. This might help the team to clarify roles.

Role motivation

As a fourth and final issue in considering roles, I suppose that nature also abhors prescriptions – human nature at least! This seems to be true in that people do not find it easy to change, particularly when they are told to change. Additionally, nature is about things in context: to understand why an animal or plant behaves as it does, one must consider its environment. Similarly, one should consider accounts of roles in context. To know that there is a prescriptive and descriptive role-profile, as in *Figure 11.1*, is not to know what is possible within that role. We therefore need to consider the motivational factors which shape a role. These include a professional's own interest in certain aspects of their job. A nurse may be skilled at counselling and be encouraged to do so by his or her manager, but find it personally difficult or demanding. As a result the nurse may avoid opportunities to counsel.

Add to this dimension the way in which clients influence staff behaviour. To illustrate, younger, less institutionalised, clients are often more responsive to nurses, making conversation more rewarding. Fraser and Cormack (1975) cite a study in which nurses were found to attempt conversations with this group of clients twice as often as with the longer-term clients. This led to a conclusion that a process of *reciprocal lethargy* occurred over time.

In a second article, Cormack and Fraser (1975) went on to address some additional factors governing the way in which the nurse's role is determined in practice. These included conflicting demands on their time (such as administration), the nature of their training, and the 'ideology' of the unit in which they worked. They presented evidence in each of these areas. For example, it appeared that the skills for which nurses were best rewarded were those that did not involve direct client care, such as administrative competence leading to promotion.

More recently, Pollock (1988) has provided a broader perspective on the motivational factors. She likened community psychiatric nursing to a theatre production:

in the face of production limitations (size of theatre, costs of time constraints etc) and the demands of sponsors, audience, critics and so on, the characters make use of the stage props and get the show on the road. The community psychiatric nurses can be likened to the characters in a play, whose title is 'The Provision of a CPN Service', the plot being individualised care (p537).

She goes on to spell out the many parallels between the production and the service (for example, 'bureaucracy'), as well as one difference. This is that actors have directors with a clear view and considerable control over how things are to be done. In contrast, nurses have to find their own solution to the constraints. Pollock's (1988) results indicate that the CPNs adopted such coping strategies as 'hit and miss' service provision (in the absence of planned care by managers) and 'playing it safe' (providing a uniform and limited service). Most fundamental of all, the nurses were unable to provide the individualised care that was central to their ideology because of insufficient resources (especially their limited available time).

Pollock's article is a welcome contribution to the discussion of the nurse's role. She has offered a helpful analogy, but more usefully she has clearly related prescriptions and descriptions by means of the motivational dimension. In this sense nurses would not be accurately perceived as 'incompetent' or 'lazy', but rather as 'failing to thrive' because of their work environment.

Interpretation

This discussion of the role of the psychiatric nurse suggests a number of potentially conflicting forces, each acting to control what is done. Some of these are highly theoretical ('prescriptions') while others are extremely practical (the 'motivational' factors). Each of these forces would represent nursing differently, with the result that conflicting messages about nursing are presented. This raises the question of what is the 'true' nature of nursing. To continue Pollock's (1988) analogy, it is as if the 'parents' of 'nursing profession' (a child with stage ambitions) had told the director of the play that their child was a veritable star just needing an opportunity to streak across the theatrical firmament. But the child actually turned up late for the first rehearsal (poor motivation, as the 'child' actually wanted to be something else), then showed little confidence and failed to impress (due to insufficient training and the raising of unrealistic expectations by the 'parents')!

To counteract this scenario, I have suggested that a detailed description (the 'role-profile'), ideally based on observation ('description'), is a sound reference point from which to consider the prescriptions and motivational perspectives. It might also be interesting to relate these forces in nursing to other mental health professions, where they are also undoubtedly present.

The material I have reviewed throughout the book, together with my own experience (including observation, co-working and discussion with nurses), tells me that these forces do produce rather different views of nursing. To put it in terms of the role profile, the 'prescriptive' force would indicate a significantly 'higher' (that is, more positive or favourable – see *Figure 11.1*) picture of the nurse, as being highly trained and utilising a wide range of skills. Descriptions of their work provided by nurses would then yield a more modest account on the profile. Finally, observations, which would inevitably take account of the motivational forces, would yield the most accurate picture.

Some of the prescriptive statements would, I suspect, hold true regardless of the perspective one took, such as '24-hour care' and the broad range of nursing duties. However, other claims or wishes expressed in response to the question we began with (that is, on the distinctive role of the mental health nurse) would not stand up to scrutiny. Indeed, from the descriptive research I have been able to locate (such as Wooff *et al.*, 1988; Pollock, 1988; Simpson, 1989) it would appear that there are essentially two 'worlds' in which nursing exists. One is 'theoretical' (the lecture hall and the journal paper) and the other is 'practical'. Sometimes they appear to coincide (as in the nurse therapy literature or the 'case studies' in the text) but more often they remain separate. Although this is unfortunate, the 'theoretical' world may serve at least two useful functions, in raising the professional status of nurses and in providing challenging and relevant goals for nursing practice. I say 'may', as it is also possible that the prescriptions will ultimately damage nursing. One way in which this could conceivably occur is if claims are made which are repeatedly refuted by the descriptive evidence. Presumably the confidence of clients, other professionals, and nurses themselves would all be undermined by such separate realities. A second way is that these prescriptions represent excessively 'challenging' goals, leading to 'failure' in the field. Both possibilities could seriously damage the morale and credibility of mental health nurses.

Conclusion

At the beginning of this book I suggested that nursing had made considerable strides during the last decade. I should now like to qualify this by saying that *theoretical* advances have made relatively huge bounds forward, while *practically* the nursing services have made strenuous efforts to keep in touch. I believe that my analysis of nursing indicates some better ways of keeping in touch, and that the psychology which informs it can become a central part of your progress as a mental health nurse. There is clearly much constructive work which can be done to shape nursing into an even more valuable and distinctive contribution to mental health promotion. This analysis will provide you with fuel and direction for that challenge.

Question for further consideration

1 I have argued that a problem solving approach can bear significant 'fruits', such as the greater professionalisation of nursing. Can you suggest additional benefits? What are the main obstacles to such developments?

2 Try to sketch out a prevention model in the form of a flowchart (as in *Figure 5.2*). Include in it all the variables which you think are important, showing how they interact with one another.

3 I have summarised Goldberg and Huxley's (1980) 'filter model', as applied to GPs. Can you set out the main filters in relation to a specific nursing consultation with a potential client? What factors in the nurse and the conduct of the interview might be important in determining whether or not the client progresses through the next filter?

4 As a nurse dedicated to improving 'social structures', what objectives might you have in your local community? How might these be pursued?

5 In *Figure 11.1* I sketched out how one could describe a nurse's distinctive role, touching on how the demands of others (such as clients and managers) would influence the profile. Try to indicate how another group of 'others' (for example, politicians or voluntary agencies) would influence the profile.

References

Bender, M. P. (1976). *Community Psychology*. London: Methuen.

Caplan, G. (1964). *Principles of Preventive Psychiatry*. New York: Basic Books.

Cormack, D. (1983). *Psychiatric Nursing Described*. Edinburgh: Churchill-Livingstone.

Cormack, D. and Fraser, D. (1975). The Nurse's Role in Psychiatric Institutions – II. *Nursing Times*, 25th December, (Occasional Paper).

Department of Health and Social Security (DHSS) (1972). *Report of the Committee on Nursing*. London: HMSO.

Fraser, D. and Cormack, D. (1975). The Nurse's role in Psychiatric Institutions – I. *Nursing Times*, 18th December, (Occasional Paper).

Goldberg, D. and Huxley, P. (1980). *Mental Illness in the Community: The Pathway to Psychiatric Care*. London: Tavistock.

Hall, J. N. (1990). Towards a psychology of caring. *British Journal of Clinical Psychology, 29*, 129–44.

Ginsberg, G. and Marks, I. (1977). Costs and benefits of behavioural psychotherapy: a pilot study of neurotics treated by nurse-therapists. *Psychological Medicine, 7*, 685–700.

Hickey, T., Rakowski, W. and Julius, M. (1988). Preventive health practices among older men and women. *Research on Ageing, 10*, 315–328.

Marks, I. M., Hallam, R. S., Connolly, J. and Philpotts, R. (1977). *Nursing in behavioural psychotherapy.* London: Royal College of Nursing.

Marks, I. M. (1985). *Psychiatric Nurse Therapists in Primary Care.* London: Royal College of Nursing.

McFarlane, J. K. (1976). A charter for caring. *Journal of Advanced Nursing, 1,* 187–196.

Newton, J. (1988). *Preventing Mental Illness.* London: Routledge.

Paykel, E. S. and Griffith, J. H. (1983). *Community Psychiatric Nursing for Neurotic Patients.* London: Royal College of Nursing.

Pollock, L. C. (1988). The work of community psychiatric nursing. *Journal of Advanced Nursing, 13,* 537–545.

Royal College of General Practitioners (1981). *Prevention of Psychiatric Disorders in General Practice* (Report from General Practice 20). London: The Royal College of General Practitioners.

Simpson, K. (1989). Community psychiatric nursing – a research-based profession? *Journal of Advanced Nursing, 14,* 274–280.

Walton, I. (1986). *The Nursing Process in Perspective: A Literature Review.* York: University Department of Social Policy and Social Work.

Ward, M. F. (1985). *The Nursing Process in Psychiatry.* Edinburgh: Churchill-Livingstone.

Wooff, K., Goldberg, D. P. and Fryers, T. (1988). The Practice of Community Psychiatric Nursing and Mental Health Social Work in Salford. *British Journal of Psychiatry, 152,* 783–792.

Further reading

Barlow, D. H., Hayes, S. C. and Nelson, R. O. (1984). *The Scientist-Practitioner.* London: Pergamon.

What Project 2000 refers to as 'knowledgeable doers', others refer to as the 'scientist-practitioner'. There is therefore much interest in this thorough going and positive book. It considers such ways of developing a research-based approach as applying single-subject studies (see Chapter 10) and testing out ideas from scientific journals in routine practice.

Brown, G. W. and Harris, T. O. (1978). *Social Origins of Depression.* London: Tavistock.

This is a fascinating and major analysis of 'prevention'. Based on a survey of women in London, Brown and Harris proposed three causal factors in depression – *provoking agents, vulnerability factors* and *symptom-formation factors.* These formed part of their psychosocial model of depression, in which life events were a large feature.

Richards, D. A. and McDonald, B. (1990). *Behavioural Psychotherapy: A Handbook for Nurses.* London: Heinemann Nursing.

In addition to reviewing the development of nurse behaviour therapy in the UK, Richards and McDonald consider recent innovations in the nurse therapist's role. These include work with those experiencing chronic pain, irritable bowel syndrome and post-traumatic stress disorder. They go on to look optimistically at the fit between nurse therapy and Project 2000, suggesting, for instance, that some behavioural skills might be taught during basic training and that nurse therapists should play a greater role in teaching students, as well as experienced colleagues (for example, CPNs). In this way, they suggest that the 'enormous potential' of nurses can be realised.

Index

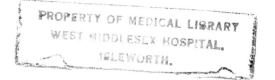